Praise for Ide

Identity Impact is an important exploration of how celebrating and uplifting diversity is essential for our health, our wellbeing, and our economic success as a community—and as a nation. Dina Proto writes with the authenticity and experience that has made her a trusted leader across LGBT, healthcare, and business organizations.

—*Justin Nelson, Co-Founder & President,*
National Gay & Lesbian Chamber of Commerce

Having been a Board certified emergency physician for 20 years, I have witnessed many facets of family and friend interactions. I have worked with and known Dina for many years and I can't think of a better person to help bring the "Identity" conversation to the forefront. Not only is she a good nurse but she is a caring, loving, and open individual. The acceptance of all people regardless of their beliefs or sexual orientation has to be started as early as possible. An open, vulnerable society will only lead to acceptance, tolerance, and love. As a father of a gay son, demonstrating our understanding and tolerance has allowed open, honest dialogue, not only in our immediate family but within our circle of friends as well.

—*Marc Jeser, DO,*
Emergency Room Medical Director

As a driving force in the LGBT business community, it's only natural for Dina to pivot her energy toward making an even bigger impact—by sharing her own journey as well as insights from years of helping people through their toughest times. Identity Impact is a thought-provoking read that's certain to spark candid conversations.

—*Dawn K. Christensen,*
LGBTQ Advocate

In Identity Impact, Proto does an exceptional job of creating a stinging awareness about the lack of available research and knowledge needed to examine how LGBTQ individuals can be impacted in their early life developmental years. Proto's analysis of the documented health trends, and statistics that touch each of the various sub cultures within the LGBTQ community, are jaw dropping. Her findings lead one to believe that once we have a solid grasp on how we can better nurture, support, and communicate with our youth, we can quite possibly find more effective ways of creating a culture of organic inclusiveness and self-love. In doing so, we can increase our levels of acceptance and appreciation for the differences of others. And we can discover how our combined perspective and life experiences contribute to how well we coexist in this melting pot of gender, cultures, lifestyles, ethnicities, and religions that all come together to make us the wonderful collective that we are. It's my sincere hope that Proto's work will rip the scab off of the festering wound of silence and shame that far too many of our LGBTQ youth are forced to live with. This book has the power to serve as the launch pad that forces us to challenge our age old beliefs and child rearing practices so that we as a society can better benefit from all the amazing talent and contributions of our LGBTQ youth.

—*Brian Martin,*
Executive Director Supplier Diversity

"What's in it for me?" As executives introduce changes to make their workplaces more LGBTQ inclusive, they are encouraged to answer this question for their non-LGBTQ employees. Identity Impact offers a helpful framework which outlines important human development milestones—namely that everyone has a gender identity and a sexual orientation. When executives lead with this reality they, along with their non-LGBTQ employees, build empathy for inequities LGBTQ people continue to endure and embrace changes that can transform a workplace climate into one that is more welcoming and inclusive for all. Give this book a read, and you'll understand how to avoid the inevitable collisions that can occur at the intersections of identity, and instead enjoy a scenic journey.

—*Rhodes Perry, CEO,*
Rhodes Perry Consulting and
Host of The Out Entrepreneur Podcast

As the mom of a self-identified bi-sexual preteen, I'm now responsible to guide and educate a child with a non-traditional identity. Guess what? I don't know how! No, I'm not talking about clean your room, share your toys, and respect your elders. That's basic across-the-board parenting. I'm talking about deeper issues with which, as a heterosexual woman, I have no experience or knowledge. That is why Identity Impact is so important. Getting information from someone who's qualified, and whose lived through difficulties with identity, is invaluable to those of us still learning. I always tell my kids they need "tools in their toolbox" to get through life (interpersonal skills, coping skills, etc.) This book gives everyone (parents, kids, educators, heath care workers, etc.) the tools that they didn't even know they needed.

—*Sherri Stupak,*
Parent

IDENTITY IMPACT

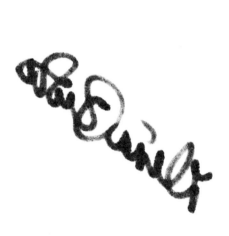

IDENTITY IMPACT

When Society's Expectations Collide with the Authentic Self

Dina Proto, RN

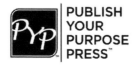

PUBLISH
YOUR
PURPOSE
PRESS

For permission requests, write to the publisher, addressed "Attention: Permissions Coordinator," at the address below.

Publish Your Purpose Press
141 Weston Street, #155
Hartford, CT 06141

The opinions expressed by the Author are not necessarily those held by Publish Your Purpose Press

Ordering Information: Quantity sales and special discounts are available on quantity purchases by corporations, associations, and others. For details, contact the publisher at the address above.

Edited by: Heather B. Habelka
Cover design by: eventart
Interior graphics: Joanna Theresa of OutLoud Graphic Designs
Printed in the United States of America.

ISBN: 978-1-946384-18-8 (print)
ISBN: 978-1-946384-19-5 (ebook)
Library of Congress Control Number: 2017955526

First edition, October 2017
Publish Your Purpose Press works with authors, and aspiring authors, who have a story to tell and a brand to build. Do you have a book idea you would like us to consider publishing? Please visit PublishYourPurposePress.com for more information.

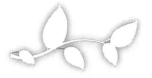

Dedication

This book is dedicated to:

Bill Thomas, for believing in us that first day we sat at your kitchen table and shared our dream to create a greeting card company for the lesbian, gay, bisexual, and transgender community, and their families and friends that was synonymous with authentic, transparent, and equitable products.

Thank you for being an incredible ally, friend, and trusted advisor who saw the void and the benefit. Your guidance and support remain the cornerstone of everything we do and not a day goes by that you are not thought of and missed immensely. Shalom my friend.

D.B.R. ~ I do and always will remember. Thank you for helping me to find my voice.

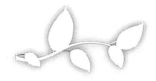

Table of Contents

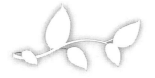

Acknowledgements

This book is a compilation of almost 50 years of impactful friendships, partnerships, and relationships. Each of which has provided me the climate and nourishment to understand my own roots and to become more healthful, hopeful, and compassionate as my own life has branched out to touch peoples' lives, whether they have been family, friend, colleague, patient, or client. Thank you for being the diversity in my garden and for shaping and molding me to be a part of the climate in the garden of society.

I want to thank my readers for taking the time to read this book and for planting the seeds for tomorrow.

I want to thank each Teazled Greeting Card & Gift customer, whether you have purchased online, in a retail chain, or in an independent store; you have been the nourishment that provided me the strength to grow and effect change.

I want to thank the Fortune 100 to Fortune 1000 companies that consistently strive to create a climate of change within their own organizations and their determination and conviction to foster a climate of change for our larger societal landscape. To the internal champions within those organizations who have been my mentors, friends, and colleagues, thank you for your gift of guidance, compassion, and encouragement to continue to touch the lives on my own tree.

To the patients and families who have allowed me to be present in your life, even for a just a moment, know that you have left a greater impact in my life than I have in yours. Thank you to my medical colleagues, friends, and mentors for sharing your chapter in my story. Maryann, thank you for being my guiding star. Know that you have all taught me to respect the potential impact I have on the people whose lives I touch. Thank you for keeping me grounded.

Thank you to Rhonda for helping me to be mindfully aware; your patience and guidance have provided me a tool of endless measure. Thank you Sam first, for answering the phone, and second, for your friendship, for asking and listening, and for understanding and then gently urging me to share, even when I was most hesitant to do so. To Sarah, Mandy, Sherri, RJ, and Ski, thank you for a lifetime of friendship and unending support, with its ups and downs, joys and sorrows, hopes and fears. I treasure each of you. To Barb, thank you for more than 10 years of love, friendship, and support on our 20-year plan. Know the you are in my heart every single day.

Thank you Mom for sharing your journey to acceptance and affirmation; and once there, for never looking back. I wouldn't change that journey, painful as it was, because without it, we wouldn't be where we are today. Thank you Dana, for working through the challenges we've faced together and for always being there, I love you more than you'll ever know, Sis. Thank you to my brother Chip for being there when I've needed you most. Thank you Pop for giving me life, loving me unconditionally, and teaching me what is most important, sempre familia.

Thank you to those of you who took the time to share your honest, candid, and at times painful life stories with me so I could illustrate the impact that identity has on each of our lives as well as the figurative point of impact and ages at which identities collide. Thank you Jenn for being a friend first, for listening, for hearing the story within that needed to be shared, and for finding the moment to gently guide me to share that story. Thank you for driving my purpose, for publishing this book, and for the scenic overlooks along the way.... even when I did want to jump. To the Publish Your Purpose Press team: Thank you Niki for keeping me organized and methodical even if I did have to use a spreadsheet! Thank you to my editor Heather for painstakingly taking my thoughts from vision to reality.

Thank you to the National Gay & Lesbian Chamber of Commerce for inviting me to have a seat at the table in 2011, for including me on the journey, and for growing me personally and professionally. I would not be who I am today without you. And to all of the other LGBTQ organizations dedicated to advocacy and change, thank you for all you do and the lives you touch.

To Nikki (Punkie), JT (Stinkmeister), Eme (Sunshine), and Anthony (Papi), thank you for being my amazingly intelligent, strong, and wise children; for making memories; and for being the catalyst that sparked the fire in me to create change through Teazled. To Alecsa, Mckenna, Ashley, and Alex thank you for being a piece of me.

And finally, I want to thank my wife Dom for being my best friend, my confidant, and the person who knows me (the real me) and loves me just the same. Thank you for countless cups of tea, treasured conversations, and humoring me. I know well the value of our love.

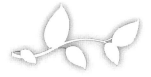

A Note from the Author

As I cultivated the information in this book, I became acutely aware that identity doesn't just happen one day. Finding one's identity is a journey; a journey that is impacted by the people and the experiences around us—like my journey to becoming an author and writing this book.

This book was written in an effort to help others understand the impact that identity can have on each of our lives and the years in which that identity formation takes place. Throughout that process, time and again my mind's eye went to a distant memory.

That memory was of my 5-year-old self and the day my parents and I moved in to our house on Hollow Road. I remember distinctly standing at a stop sign two houses down at the intersection of Hollow and Hope—the intersection where I would meet two sisters. At the age of 5, I had no idea the impact that would have on my identity. Neither did they.

Fast forward more than 40 years, when I was faced with selecting an image for the cover. I had to consider what message I wanted the cover to convey. It was critical that the image would connect the reader to the impact of the information contained inside.

What makes this image so important?

The truth is, it's important because it's real. It's real in the sense that the intersection of Hope and Hollow, really does exist—both literally and figuratively. And the oak tree, it's really there too. That intersection depicts the choice in my own life to choose to be full of Hope rather than continuing to be Hollow. And, I personally believe that not everyone is given the perspective and visual representation I've been given to see that intersection in their own lives. Sometimes we need the person who has taken the journey before us to pave the way. It is my hope that I can be that for others.

So how did I get that photograph you ask? I've been told it's a rarity to have childhood friends one remains close with throughout their life. And yet, that is my reality. I can thank Sherri Stupak for answering the call of an old childhood friend, for taking the time to see my vision, and for helping me to share a piece of my identity. Thank you for being the eyes at my intersection and helping others to see what it looks like when you turn the corner from Hollow to Hope.

—Dina

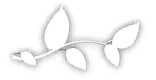

Foreword

So there I am, running around—late, as usual.

I needed cards for my moms (no, that isn't a typo) for Mothers' Day.

But, as to be expected, there were no cards that read "To My Two Moms on Mothers' Day."

Dammit.

So I grabbed a couple of cards that more or less expressed some semblance of the sentiment I wished to express and proceeded to cross out and alter the cards as I saw fit.

I had one for my birth mom and one for my dad mom, Dom for short (amazingly this nickname has stuck over the years). It was this incident that incited an (initially jovial) conversation about creating our own cards to fill a very real need our family had identified.

How does that bring us here to this book, you ask?

My mother, in all her whirlwind ways, identified a greater need linked to the lack of greeting cards designated to "subcultures" as it were. Our society at large has moved forward in many ways, but an understanding of how identities develop with any breadth and depth has been sadly marginalized.

This book is a way to help friends, family, and professionals bridge the gap between what we think we know and what is.

—*Nichole Marie Scheidt*

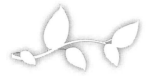

Preface

THE IMPACT LEFT BY THE LEAVES ON MY OWN TREE

My life has indeed been a crazy journey … I've been blessed with incredible scenic overlooks. Some have been tucked back, out of the purview of others, and some have been visible for all to see. Some have been at the edge of a cliff and some have been on plateaus in the high desert.

Each overlook has provided me the ability and the responsibility to impact my own identity. And each has spurred me to impact the identity of others, whether I realized it at the time or not.

Even the journey to write this book.

When I first began, I thought I was writing a brochure to justify to retailers why they should carry my company's greeting cards for the LGBTQ (lesbian, gay, bisexual, transgender, queer) community and just how many people needed the products we provided. Silly me.

Instead, I emerged with what I discovered were a multitude of health issues caused by invalidation of one's identity and the lack of education and awareness within the healthcare system to meet the needs of the LGBTQ community. That's what happens when a nurse sets out to justify a rationale. I was attempting to justify the rationale that not only did the more than 9 million LGBTQ Americans deserve greeting cards readily available to them, but so did the 87% of Americans who knew and loved them.

So, I began to write. Little did I know that this particular overlook would be the catalyst for my own self-discovery along the way.

Little did I really understand my own Identity Impact.

Until now.

I'm wondering if you will notice any similarities (or differences) in the pages that lie ahead, whether in relation to my own life's journey, the metaphors I use, or the medical knowledge I impart, or the real-life scenarios that I share. While I do admittedly share some of my own family experience and dysfunction, it wouldn't be nearly as entertaining if I removed the root of all the "fun" in dysfunction.

The truth is, we all struggle through stages of growth and development. We all struggle with some measure of conflict resolution and, at some point in our lives, we learn the virtue that has eluded us.

However, those along the LGBTQ continuum experience an additional layer of development as well as stages of grieving (by themselves and their families) that further adds impact to their personal identity, development, and coping mechanisms. Those coping mechanisms can then culminate into health issues at higher rates than our heterosexual peers.

Another unintentional discovery along this journey has been the realization that the average age to identify bares out to be about 11 years of age, yet many seem to struggle with that process for an additional 10 to 15 years before finding peace in a landscape that allows them to flourish.

This book will help to provide insight that the very people in our lives trained with the ability to mold and shape us to prepare to be adults; are they themselves ill-prepared to understand and guide the growth and development of those within the LGBTQ community due to lack of research, best practices, and consistent education requirements for professionals afforded through our current processes and knowledge dissemination.

Our current cultural practices perpetuate treating health complications *after* they occur as opposed to providing education that can *prevent* health complications.

In fact, several of the real-life experiences shared reveal a lack of perceived positive impact by parents, healthcare workers, psychologists, educators, media, businesses, and church or political leaders.

For example, Alicia, a 20-to-24-year-old trans woman was introduced to me early in her senior year by her healthcare provider. He wanted to provide her with appropriate care and was acutely aware he was not familiar with the resources available to support her (we happened to know each other and he was aware of my work in the community). He was ahead of the curve.

For me personally, that single life (or leaf) that represents Alicia on my own tree, has provided immeasurable impact that Alicia may not come to understand for many years. I remember having her and her parents to our home for dinner shortly after we met. Her parents were struggling with their own thoughts and feelings and their own set of fears, as well as trying to figure out how to navigate the relationship dynamics in their immediate and extended family. Alicia was struggling with how owning her identity would impact and potentially change the relationship she had with her brothers. Both Alicia and her parents had fears about college campus safety, dorm living arrangements, and safety in general.

I will always remember the gift Alicia gave to me by allowing me to witness her own journey after she came out to her friends the last day of school her senior year. We set a girls day to get our hair and nails done, get her ears pierced, and shop for a new wardrobe. We finished it off with a celebratory sushi dinner. I remember feeling both honor and sadness at the same time. I had watched her face light up as she picked up a light blue blouse and said she had "always wanted one," and in that single defining moment, I felt sadness that her own mother had missed that piece of her journey. I am so very happy that she and her family have transitioned to a better place together. And I watch in awe as she has become an advocate in her own right and continues to pay it forward.

My ask is that, as you read the pages that lie ahead, please be aware of your own verbal and nonverbal messaging to others. If you are in a position to impact other people's lives, be mindful of the biases you come to the table with, the words and descriptors you use, and the nonverbal messages you send both intentionally and unintentionally.

Look at the landscape around you and choose to create a climate of acceptance and affirmation for all of the identities of the leaves on your own branches and on the branches of others. And remember that we collectively reap the seeds we sow.

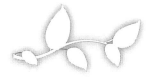

Removing Sex from the Identity Equation

"I speak for the trees, for the trees have no tongues."

—Dr. Seuss, The Lorax

As a registered nurse, I have spent the last 23 years learning and honing my nursing skills. And do I have skills! I can take your vital signs, start an IV, medicate you for pain, do CPR, and assess your physical injuries and illnesses to name a few. But that's not why you would want me as your nurse. Those skill sets can be taught to *anyone*.

You want me as your nurse because I excel at looking at the big picture; analyzing systems if you will. I pay attention to detail, the things people say both verbally and nonverbally. You want me as your nurse because I remain calm under pressure. I'm a communicator, educator, critical thinker, and planner. I'm flexible and compassionate.

You want me as your nurse because I advocate for you, even when I may personally struggle with your choices. I advocate for you because I want you to respect me when the shoe is on the other foot. And make no mistake, advocacy is an uphill battle 90%

of the time because we all think we have the answer and that we're on the right side.

It's those nursing skills that pushed me to look at the big picture in a way no other has.

I was surprised to find that since the late 80s, we as a society have begun to intentionally take a closer look at the LGBTQ community—by first attempting to remove the stigma of the attachment of a medical diagnosis to people who were something other than heterosexual. From that point forward, there has been a focus on both HIV and AIDS, followed by increased awareness of not only social disparities that exist, but also work and health disparities. Where there was once little information and insight, we have begun to realize we need to dig deeper, gather more research, evaluate more statistics, and then use that information to determine how we can change outcomes.

Each and every aspect is vital to moving forward.

However, in looking at the big picture, the "system," if you will, there is a disconnect between the research that has been obtained and when that research is disseminated. Although more research will be needed to continue to gain greater insight, a significant barrier remains to being able to effectively accomplish that statistical insight.

That barrier is identification.

I don't mean walking through town trying to label each person.

You see, there are no set external indicators for determining or identifying someone as LGBTQ. There is no visual cue.

Instead, our current process and system rely on self-identification and sharing of that knowledge. So much so that the statistical information we *do* have relies *solely* on those of us who chose to share our identity publicly, those of us who voluntarily respond to surveys, and those who live our lives "out" in advocacy.

Until such time that we begin to understand the impact personal identity has on each of us as well as the stigma we project on those who do not conform to the perceived norm of heterosexuality, we will continue to struggle to gain true understanding of the number of people, the impact made on the lives of those people, and ultimately, the impact made on society.

Multiple organizations have researched, gathered, and publicly posted their findings whether they impact social, economic, financial, emotional, and physical aspects of the LGBTQ community. What is missing is looking at the systemic issues that prevail and the point in one's life where we can affect the most significant change.

That point is the true Identity Impact.

The best way I can explain it is by using the following example: Imagine you're a runner.

You've been running for years and put a lot of wear and tear on your right knee. Your doctor has suggested you have a knee replacement and you have reluctantly agreed, because your hope is that you can run again at some point shortly after surgery and be better than you have been in recent years.

It's surgery day ... you check in at the local hospital and meet the nurses, surgeon, anesthesiologist (the doctor/nurse who sedates you so you don't feel the process or remember it). You sign your consents, your IV is started, and away you go.

After several hours, you're awake, you're in a fair amount of pain, but you can move your right knee (which completely surprises you). But you can't for the life of you figure out why your left knee is in excruciating pain! No, they didn't. They couldn't have. They replaced your *left* knee instead of your *right* knee!

Now, not only are you in pain, but they didn't even fix the knee that was bothering you! You won't be able to return to running when you thought because you still have to heal from this surgery and then have the correct *right* knee replaced. And, on top of it, you used the vacation time from work you had to save up for this surgery, you've got insurance co-pays, and you need to go through it all over again!

That, my friend, is a "sentinel event." An unanticipated outcome of events.[1]

It's a story we've probably heard, mocked, or laughed at because it didn't happen to us personally and we probably thought something along the lines of: How could they be so dumb?

Well, while we're all busy thinking and chuckling at the thought that something like that could happen, the hospital and its staff are busy analyzing what happened and why.

What system can be improved to prevent that outcome and negative impact from happening?

You see, when you don't know that something is broken, you can't fix it.

You see, when you don't know that something is broken, you can't fix it.

But when you know, you have the knowledge *and* the responsibility to help prevent that sentinel event or negative outcome from happening in the future.

But when you know, you have the knowledge *and* the responsibility to help prevent that sentinel event or negative outcome from happening in the future.

As you undoubtedly know, our society stands very clearly to the "left" or to the "right" of LGBTQ issues, often

---

[1]Sentinel event. (2017, August 20). Retrieved September 15, 2017, from https://en.wikipedia.org/wiki/Sentinel_event

attempting to define an individual based on outward expression of self—as opposed to allowing one to define their identity on their own terms.

So what does that mean?

Many of our own perceptions or personal biases (in either direction) are based on the information we have at any given moment, our personal roots, the climate in which we live, what we were taught either in school or at home, and our personal experiences.

The goal of this book is not to tell you that your beliefs are wrong.

Nurses are taught in Nursing 101 not to make judgments, but rather to accept each person or patient at wherever they are in their own journey (and, trust me, that is not always easy!). The idea of meeting a person where they are rather than trying to bring them to our expectation for our own life cannot be exclusive to nursing.

We have far too many "sentinel events" within the LGBTQ community. Those sentinel events are the result of lack of acceptance as something other than the preconceived societal norm of heterosexual relationships and the gender roles associated with them. What I mean by that is, as a society, we try to define or categorize people using two specific columns (male or female) and the cultural roles associated with each of them.

Things like depression, suicide, homelessness, drug addiction, risky sex behaviors, isolation, anxiety, obesity, diabetes, coronary artery disease, stroke, congestive heart failure, HIV/AIDS, Hepatitis B & C, sexually transmitted diseases (STDs), intimate partner violence, substance abuse, lack of healthcare treatment, sustainable occupations and careers, inadequate housing, and self fulfillment are all signs and symptoms of a larger process at work.

They themselves may indeed become the "sentinel event" for which no one is preparing.

Each of these issues is impacted by and ultimately impacts our society either on an emotional or financial level or both. Before you can begin to address the sentinel events and the signs and symptoms that they're just around the corner, you must first look at the root cause.

I believe the root cause of these sentinel events, which are commonly associated with the LGBTQ community, are not the mere *being* LGBTQ, but more so the way our current society projects our gender role (often prior to birth) and how attempting to live up to that projected expectation can have lasting effects on the individual and society.

I believe the root cause of these sentinel events, which are commonly associated with the LGBTQ community, are not the mere *being* LGBTQ, but more so the way our current society projects our gender role (often prior to birth) and how attempting to live up to that projected expectation can have lasting effects on the individual and society.

It is our identity, not our sexuality, that has the greatest impact.

It is our identity, not our sexuality, that has the greatest impact.

My hope is that you will come to understand your own roots and those of the people who are part of your community so we can all thrive in the same landscape together, full of hope rather than a hollow existence.

Each of us can have either a positive or negative impact on the greater system and ultimately the "sentinel events" affecting the LGBTQ community. *Identity Impact* is designed specifically to help you not only understand your own roots, bias, and personal impact, but to provide you with insight into the ways we individually and collectively impact identity.

To help you accomplish that, I've systematically and intentionally removed the idea of sex or "intercourse" from the conversation (at least initially). I did that so you can begin to see the entire system without personal bias (or at least understanding your own personal bias) and its ultimate impact. The best place is to start at the root.

To do that, let's look at one's sense of personal identity and the summation of parts.

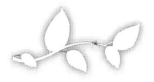

The Sum is Equal to All Its Parts

"Nothing of me is original. I am the combined effort of everyone I've ever known."

—Chuck Palahniuk

Merriam Webster defines *identity* as "the condition of being the same with something described or asserted; feeling that you share and understand the problems or experiences of another person: the act of identifying *with* someone."[2]

If, however, you were to look up the word "identity" in a medical dictionary, the definition varies slightly to be more inclusive: "The summation of a person's internalized history of relationship with objects, his or her social role, and his or her perception of both; the experience of 'I.'"[3]

Let's take a moment to take inventory of your identity.

---

[2]Identity. (n.d.). Retrieved March 16, 2017, from https://www.merriam-webster.com/dictionary/identity

[3]Identity. (n.d.). Retrieved March 16, 2017, from https://www.merriam-webster.com/dictionary/identity#medicalDictionary

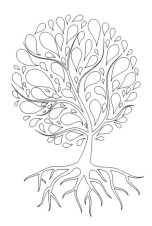

Grab a pencil and blank sheet of paper (or download the template I've created at dinaproto.com/template).

First, draw the roots of a tree.

On those roots, write down words that describe who you are, the very things that make you, you and form *your* sense of identity:

Are you male or female?
Are you a parent or child?
A sister or a brother?
A mother or a father?
A grandmother or a grandfather?
An aunt or an uncle?
A friend or a lover?
What is your profession?
What interests/hobbies do you enjoy?

How many ways did you choose to describe yourself?
What words did you choose and why did you choose them?
Did you include words about your family of origin? Ethnicity? Culture? Faith?

All those words you chose to write down about your roots are *your* identity.

As you can see, our "roots" or identity are multifaceted.

Remember what we learned in math all those years ago?

The sum is equal to all its parts.

So too, is identity.

Now take your pencil and fill in the landscape—

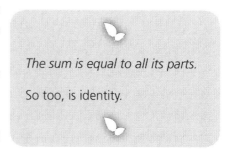

the grass, hills, and valleys—around your roots. Write down things your roots need to grow (think: water, food, shelter, etc.).

Next, I'd like you to go ahead and draw your trunk. Your trunk can be as skinny or as fat as you'd like. (This isn't an activity indicating how healthy you are).

If the trunk is the main stem from where all branches of the tree grow, we need to consider its function in life: to support the growth of all branches and leaves by providing sustenance. The bark is the "skin" of the tree that protects the inner living tissue of the tree. That bark or skin can take many forms and, regardless of the type of tree, all trees have rings and life cycles.

Somewhere in years past, we learned in science class that, "Tree rings grow under the bark and that the bark is pushed out while the tree is growing. The inner part of a growth ring is formed early in the growing season, when growth is fast it is known as early wood. The outer portion is the late wood, and is denser than early wood."[4]

---

[4]Growth ring. (2017, August 11). Retrieved September 03, 2017, from https://simple.wikipedia.org/wiki/Growth_ring

We also learned that the trunk of a tree contains both its "heartwood" and "sapwood."

According to sactree.com, a tree's "heartwood" forms as a result of aging in normal compartments of a tree. "Heartwood" cannot respond to injury but it does discolor.[5] However, "sapwood" responds to injury and forms a natural resistance to decay. If you're sensing my reference to the emotional damage that can be caused during those early stages of development, you're definitely paying attention.

sactree.com also goes on to say that "false heartwood" is a central column of discoloration that occurs as a young tree matures, when many branches die and are shed even though there may be no decay. Discoloration that takes place in the early stages of decay after a tree is injured is not true heartwood, but it can keep heartwood from forming."[6]

The bad news is that we, as a society, are creating identities with "false heartwood" that result in hollow adults.

The good news is that I actually recalled something useful from science class. Sister John Ann would be impressed.

The bad news is that, sometimes the insight we needed during our own early growing season, isn't available to us until we're in that "late wood" stage ourselves.

And by then, we're dense.

What I mean by saying we're "dense" as we grow older is that it can take us longer to process information, not due to lack of intelligence, but rather due to the tons of thoughts that fly through our heads as we struggle to understand something we haven't

---

[5]The Anatomy of a Tree. (2002, February 27). Retrieved March 15, 2017, from http://www.sactree.com/assets/files/greenprint/toolkit/c/huntsvilleTreeGuide.pdf

[6]The Anatomy of a Tree. (2002, February 27). Retrieved March 15, 2017, from http://www.sactree.com/assets/files/greenprint/toolkit/c/huntsvilleTreeGuide.pdf

personally had to deal with and then, the only way we seem to receive that information is with a jaded mind that our society and culture have taught us.

But we're working past that here.

If you're that younger tree in your faster growth season, go ahead and draw how many rings you have. If you're that older tree in the slower season of growth, then you're a little thicker in the middle with more rings (be happy they're not wrinkles!)

Go ahead and write your name on the trunk.

Those rings are all the ways in which we grow and change on the inside. The bark, on the other hand, is the piece of us the outside world sees. Sometimes, that "bark" appears healthy and sometimes that "bark" is scarred.

My point here is that you get to decide how the outside world sees you. You do that every day when you get up, shower, and dress for work or play. You show the world your bark, but the question is: Are you hollow inside or full of hope? Is what you show the world who you really are?

Next, I want you to draw the sun and, on the rays of the sun, I want you to write down all of the elements that influence how you grow. Parents? Friends? Educators? Doctors? Media?

Don't forget there are many factors that influence your growth like climate, weather, rain, temperature, pH, nutrition, carbon dioxide, and sunspots. That doesn't mean you can't be a tree that is strong, healthy, and beautiful, just that

> You show the world your bark, but the question is: Are you hollow inside or full of hope? Is what you show the world who you really are?

you've weathered a few storms and have survived in spite of your climate.

The next facet of growth for your tree is the formation of branches and ultimately leaves. If you've identified yourself as a tree that flowers or produces fruit, your next growth stage is the formation of a union graft.

According to Dan Gill, *The Times-Picayune* garden columnist, "Grafting is a common horticulture technique. It's an efficient method of propagation that produces offspring genetically identical to the original plant."[7] Okay, clearly having offspring that are exactly like the original could be positive or negative, but I'll let you draw your own conclusion about that.

It's at the "union graft," the point of intersection between the two trees that we see the intersection of identity taking shape.[8] Grafting is done to combine the best characteristics of two trees. You see, one of the trees is the root stock that provides the lower portion of the tree trunk and roots. The other tree is the scion that the upper portion (the flowers, leaves or fruit) eventually grow from.

According to thepsruce.com in *Special Growing Considerations for Grafted Plants* "You have to be careful when planting grafted plants. If the graft joint is buried underground, the rootstock can sprout its own top growth or the scion can send down its own

---

[7]Dan Gill, The Times-Picayune garden columnist. (2015, March 05). How, when and why plants are grafted. Retrieved April 18, 2017, from http://www.nola.com/homegarden/index.ssf/2015/03/how_when_and_why_plants_are_gr.html

[8]Graft union | Definition of graft union in English by Oxford Dictionaries. (n.d.). Retrieved March 15, 2017, from https://en.oxforddictionaries.com/definition/graft_union

roots. When that happens, you lose the characteristics selected for when the plant was grafted."[9]

As a parent, this process causes me to consider my own children and what is buried underground for each of them. Did I give them what they needed to sprout their own top growth? It's the impact at this intersection of the union graft that is so powerful. And that power, my friend, can be beautiful or ugly.

---

[9]Dan Gill, The Times-Picayune garden columnist. (2015, March 05). How, when and why plants are grafted. Retrieved April 18, 2017, from http://www.nola.com/homegarden/index.ssf/2015/03/how_when_and_why_plants_are_gr.html

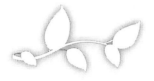

Identity: Yours, Mine and How We Impact Each Other

N
ow that you've formed your union graft, go ahead and draw those branches as long and as wide as you'd like.

On those branches, I want you to write down the relationships in your life. What are the relationships that you value? On my branches, I'd write down things like: romantic (my wife), family (immediate and extended), and friendships (professional, faith-based, community, or civic-based).

Onto, perhaps, the most precious part of your tree.

I want you to *really* think about this next part carefully.

Go ahead and take a few minutes to think of *all* the lives you touch every single day from each of your roots and list those lives on your leaves. You can use individual names. You can use relationships as well. Remember, if your branches are the ones that are long and wide, you've got a lot of lives, I mean leaves, to fill in.

If you're not sure where to start, I can share a few of mine: my wife, each of my four children, my siblings, family members, and friends to name a few. But those are the obvious answers right? How about as a nurse: each patient I've ever taken care of, each family member who I sat bedside, each co-worker (regardless of what they do). How about as an entrepreneur: each customer (potential and current) and each business I've encountered. As a community leader: each entrepreneur I've met, advocated for, and mentored. The same is true at my church, the Chamber of Commerce I founded in Las Vegas, and the National Gay and Lesbian Chamber of Commerce of which I'm a part.

FACTORS THAT INFLUENCE GROWTH

The last thing I want you to draw in are the elements that affect your growth.

This part of the exercise reminds me of when my wife and I were getting married. The minister gave us one of those wrought iron wall hangings and referred to it throughout the ceremony. The wall hanging was a vase filled with two skinny branches or twigs. What she shared with us was that we were each a branch or twig resting in the same vase and how, over time, our individual roots would be nurtured and begin to join as one; ultimately strengthening our tree.

And, over time, our tree would grow in girth (I didn't think she meant we'd gain weight, but apparently all married couples are prone to that!) and form branches that would reach out to touch the lives of others. Those branches would bend and sway over the years, continuing to produce branches and leaves the likes of which had never been seen. And that tree, it would start with our individual roots.

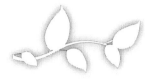

What Kind of Tree Are You?

"The reward for conformity is that everybody likes you except yourself."

—Rita Mae Brown, author of Rubyfruit Jungle

What kind of tree did you choose to be? Are you an oak or maple tree because they're strong, a willow because they're flexible, or did you choose a cherry or apple tree because they help to sustain life by providing sustenance? All of those qualities have value.

> *As long as you're tall.*
> *As long as you have a sturdy trunk.*
> *As long as your leaves are green, almond-shaped, and shiny.*
> *Wait, you're not happy with this direction? What's wrong?*
> *You didn't want almond-shaped leaves?*
> *I'm sorry, trees with sturdy trunks have almond-shaped leaves.*
> *You wanted purple leaves instead of green?*
> *I'm sorry, only trees with thin trunks get purple leaves.*
> *Did you just question your identity?*

How could you not? I did indeed tell you, after all, you could be anything you wanted to be—as long as you have a sturdy trunk and green, almond-shaped leaves.

How did what I just did impact the way you felt about your tree? Your ego? Your sense of self?

Your identity?

I'm wondering what you're feeling. I'm wondering if you're questioning why I asked you what was important to you when, in the end, I didn't really care.

By ignoring or invalidating what you envisioned for yourself as a tree and forcing you to conform to *my* ideal of a tree, I'm inadvertently saying that you're not good enough the way you are.

The truth is you are. And, I do care.

The truth is, you are all of the parts of your tree that make you, you.

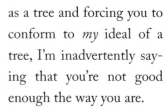

By ignoring or invalidating what you envisioned for yourself as a tree and forcing you to conform to *my* ideal of a tree, I'm inadvertently saying that you're not good enough the way you are.

Just like I am all of the parts of my tree that make me, me. That doesn't mean that your tree is more or less valuable than my tree, you're just a different tree.

To carry that one step further, we're both trees in the same forest with lots of other trees. Some of the trees are like you and some of those trees are like me. And some of those trees are a blending of our trees. And each of our trees *can* and *do* grow in that same forest or garden at different rates and seasons. It might even be that your tree can provide shelter for my tree when the weather is harsh. And, at the end of the seasons, when your growth is slower, maybe, just maybe, it's my tree that provides your sun-damaged leaves with carbon dioxide and nutrients to leave new seeds and growth behind.

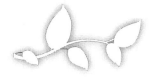

Personal Identity

"In the social jungle of human existence, there is no feeling of being alive without a sense of identity."

—Erik Erikson

When I began writing *Identity Impact,* I was repeatedly drawn to the image of a tree.

I assumed this was because my wife and I have made the image of a tree part of our lives and our business. In fact, we chose the tree as the basis of the logo for our greeting card and gift company years ago.

In retrospect, the image of a tree is more than a logo, it's a part of me, my identity.

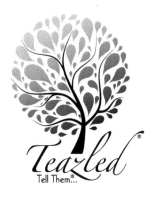

At its roots, the tree indicates my own personal identity; my roles as a daughter, sister, wife, mother, nurse, lesbian, entrepreneur, and community leader; and how they together formed my sense of me (my trunk) and the lives of the people I had hoped our greeting cards would touch.

I should probably backtrack here a bit to give you a little personal history.

Dom (that's the name our kids, family, and friends gave my wife) and I decided to open Teazled Greeting Cards and Gifts in the spring of 2011. I had spent 18 months recovering from a bilateral mastectomy and during that time I reflected on how I was spending my days. What chapter was I writing in my life's journal? Although I had been a wife, mother, and nurse for many years, I was aware that my own growth pattern had been impacted by climate, weather, rain, temperature, pH, nutrition, carbon dioxide, and sunspots. When you're given another season to enjoy, you make different choices and decisions with new insight you didn't have before.

I decided nursing wasn't the only way I could nurture others and I wanted to leave not just a footprint in the forest or garden, but I wanted to plant seeds to cultivate for future growth.

I wanted my life to have had meaning and positive impact. Fortunately for me, Dom has always been very supportive of my harebrained ideas (including this book). When Dom and I decided to plant the Teazled seed and open in August of 2011, all we had to rely on to prove our business model was our personal journey as lesbians and our knowledge as nurses about the importance of communication in relationships and the aftermath that occurs when people don't effectively and openly communicate what they're feeling. You see, sometimes we have the same wants and fears and express them in different ways.

Our family had waited for the availability of greeting cards to give to each other. We realized if we couldn't readily find cards to communicate with our family, neither could other LGBTQ families. Our children wanted us to fix that. We knew communication was the key to maintaining any of our most valued relationships. Our "leaves," if you get my drift.

We set out to learn all we could about the greeting card industry. We also set out to learn all we could about the LGBTQ community and just how many lives are really affected by the coming out process and living authentically. We wanted to plant a seed that would one day become a living, breathing legacy, touching more lives than we could ever imagine.

It's probably most important to explain here why the tree is so very important and how it represents our commitment. Yes, those twigs or branches from our ceremony were the foundation that planted the seed. And yes, those individual saplings grafted together to create our identity.

It is Teazled that forms the base of the trunk, our strength in providing the LGBTQ community greeting cards and gifts today. And it is our knowledge and insight in to the LGBTQ community that provides our strength to continue to branch out and touch the lives (or leaves) on the Teazled tree.

What we once thought would be an online greeting card company has had many life cycles, each encouraged by the lives we support. Time and again we've received requests to be more readily available. Time and again, customers asked for us to be in local stores. Their requests have been the nourishment we needed to grow.

In the early years, we *may* have secretly watched customers read our cards in grocery store aisles, knowing we had accomplished what we were once told would never happen. Imagine two nurses learning the ins and outs of greeting card design, UPC codes, wholesale, and retail!

We actually had people tell us that we should sell our cards in adult stores, but we just couldn't imagine suggesting our parents or children go to an adult store for a Mothers' Day or Christmas card!

We eventually found our way in to a grocery store chain and then, in April 2015, we opened our own brick and mortar location for "Teazled Greeting Cards & Gifts" in Downtown Las Vegas. With little to no advertising, we had customers come in from all over the country and the globe saying, "I can't find any cards like these in my city" or "Can you open one of these in my city?"

Talk about a humbling and powerful experience!

One of the most interesting things I learned from working in our retail space was just how many shoppers stumbled in to the store, not knowing who we were or what we did, and ultimately, shared their own family coming out stories (their own and their loved ones), and felt like they were in a safe space to do so. I remember one night in particular when a group of about 15 youth ended up sitting on the floor inside our 170 square foot "container" store telling us their stories and what the cards and products meant to them.

I can't tell you the number of parents, grandparents, siblings, and friends who said they had waited for what seemed like an eternity before their loved one "came out."

I can't express the humbling feeling knowing that people sought us out as a safe place to share their identity stories. Or the joy of an 86-year-old grandmother driving an hour because she heard we had cards and gifts for her granddaughter who was becoming her grandson. She wanted to show her support, she just didn't know how. What an honor to be a resource for other families experiencing the same challenges, hopes, and fears as our family!

Time and time again I watched people read the greeting cards, tears streaming from their eyes. Time and time again people commented, "I wish I had this when ..."

So, when I say the image of a tree is part of my identity, it is indeed true. I am the sum of all of my parts, all of the things that make me, me. Just as you are the sum of all of your parts that make you, you.

You see, it's simple to draw a picture. I know I'm not the only one who's gone to one of those wine and canvas parties where a local artist teaches each of the party goers to paint the same image.

When Dom and I went to one, the artist had us draw a tree! Don't think for one second that "coincidence" was lost on me!

It's easy to craft an image when someone is guiding you and telling you what to do. And even though that artist is painstakingly showing each person exactly how to paint those roots, trunks, branches, leaves, and flowers, no two paintings come out exactly the same. And there isn't one in the bunch that's perfect, not even to the painter.

Over the years, my own tree has seen several seasons of change.

We all have seasons of change, and it's a season of change for society.

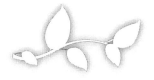

Getting to the Root

"It's not about what it is, it's about what it can become."

—Dr. Seuss, The Lorax

I've found that as I've continued my quest to identify a single point that our society can agree has the same merit and value, I've searched for that common point in our lives that we can go back to where we weren't jaded with the scars that formed our trunks, but rather where we experienced new growth at the same rate.

In my own journey to self discovery and acceptance, I have come to realize that we, as a society, have a tendency to negate the power of individuality long before children even know what that means, let alone who they are. It is easy to project our acceptance or displeasure with adolescents and adults who make choices that are contrary to those we would have made for them. So, at what point do we, as a society, mutually agree that each individual is valued just as they are, as opposed to how we perceive they should be?

I thought I could do enough research to show that there is indeed value in each "tree" or person to cultivate growth.

I even thought that maybe I could help others see that, down deep at our very roots, we all have the same basic needs, regardless of the various ways we set out to achieve those needs.

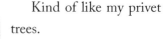

At what point do we, as a society, mutually agree that each individual is valued just as they are, as opposed to how we perceive they should be?

Kind of like my privet trees.

I have two in the back yard, each placed prominently in the right and left corners.

The tree on the left is at a slightly higher gradient than the tree on the right and is shaded by our butterfly bush and fan palm tree. That privet on the left is vibrant in its own right and grows taller every year. The tree on the right, however, is shaded by our orange tree and flowering oleander. But for some reason, nothing I do has helped that privet tree to grow. Now, that orange tree and flowering oleander provide massive beauty as well. But the privet by those trees, although it has strength and beauty in its own right, continues to struggle through each season. The seedlings and soil were exactly the same. I watered them and fed them the same. I pruned them the same. And they couldn't be more different. And yet, the same.

See where I'm going with this?

As I'm writing this, I'm actually sitting in the back yard looking at them and I'm struck by how my example of growth seemed to naturally present a position that was clearly to the far "right" and far "left." And, sure as I sit here, it's the redwood ash smack dab in the middle of the yard that is providing me shade and shelter from the scorch of the sun. It has the same trunk girth as both the privets and was planted at the same time in the same soil.

But there are more branches that extend further and, although the leaves are similar in size and shape, they are more plentiful and closely situated. Both types of trees lose their leaves in the harsh of winter. But that redwood ash in the middle of the yard provides shade that far exceeds the shade of either privet—and the leaves turn an amazingly beautiful fire red in the fall.

Even stranger still, is how our society views the growth and development, and ultimately lives, of our children. And the means we will go to in order to force a union graft that may ultimately bury that intersection or joint and, in effect, destroy the very characteristics we had hoped would develop in the first place. It's time to transition now from that image of a tree for a little while. But we'll back to nature, nonetheless.

Let's head back to school, the horticulture school that is. That's where the specialists, the horticulturists, and farmers learn how to plant, grow, and prune all the plants and trees to provide food, shelter, and products for us.

In *our* world, that would be the equivalent of psychologists and therapists who spend years learning and theorizing about the growth and development of us as people.

Now remember, it's not just the horticulturist or farmer who learns the details, but many of us (regardless of our career paths) learn the basics at some point so we can tend to our own yard, garden, or (if we're really lucky) a larger piece of landscape.

It turns out that multiple career paths (not just psychology and medicine) all learn the same stages of development and each of those careers apply the information differently, depending on their role and identity. A quick Google search (even by those of us who are technologically challenged) produces a pretty extensive list of careers that use them. Check out degrees or curriculum for teaching, social work, art/design, business, engineering, hospitality, law, technology, marketing, communication and media, retail, finance, and manufacturing.

I also found that while we all focus on our own little space and role (identity), our larger whole (society) defines what "trees" are tended to and which ones are perceived to have less value or impact.

Moving away from the metaphor: it would seem as though society at large determines value and pertinence of individuals and groups alike based on outdated ideologies, family structures, and cultural ideals that no longer mirror the image of our present-day society.

Enter the "trees" that have the ability to transform the present landscape. Landscape without variation eventually becomes desolate and barren (think Dr. Seuss's *The Lorax*).

Enter the "trees" that are not just privets but the orange tree, the oleander, the palm, and the butterfly.

Regardless of the diverse qualities of the tree (internal and external), each has value and purpose in the landscape. That diversity in our culture and society, by the same token, takes many forms. Sometimes it's cultural, ethnic, spiritual, and political. Sometimes that diversity is visible in our external appearance (seen by both others and by ourselves). Other times still, that diversity is internal in terms of who and why we love.

For many of you reading this, you are already familiar with those who are part of the LGBTQ community.

For others, it's like walking through an English Garden when you're used to the landscape in the Mojave Desert. It's important to understand that the words, and sometimes letters, used to identify oneself as part of a particular group are only one single aspect of identity.

Remember: The sum is equal to all of its parts.

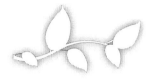

Defining Stereotypes

"We can spend our lives letting the world tell us who we are. Sane or insane. Saints or sex addicts. Heroes or victims. Letting history tell us how good or bad we are. Letting our past decide our future. Or we can decide for ourselves. And maybe it's our job to invent something better."

—Chuck Palahniuk

I identify as a lesbian, yes.

That identity *is not* about a sexual act. It's about an aspect of me, of who I am. It's about the person who fulfills my need for emotionally intimate love.

The letters LGBTQ are *part* of an identity, letters many people use to identify themselves as part of a larger group outside the socially and culturally accepted heterosexual identity.

Those letters *do not* define all that embodies someone who identifies as part of the LGBTQ community nor do they validate a "lifestyle" or stereotype.

Think about that for a minute.

If you don't know someone who is LGBTQ, you may be inclined to believe that the very nature of "being LGBTQ" includes a life of drug and alcohol abuse, sexually risky behavior, lack of education, financial instability, homelessness, STDs, mental illness, etc. Although, you could be of the mindset that the LGBTQ "lifestyle" applies to everyone *but* your loved one, that perception happens too.

A word of caution here: Please don't make the assumption that you can identify someone by their outward expression of self as anywhere on the LGBTQ continuum. You know what they say when you "assume" *and*, since we're each as unique as the sum of our personal identities, that sure would be a lot of stereotypes to learn about!

Here's where the nurse in me comes out. These "lifestyle" descriptors or stereotypes don't define those in the LGBTQ community, but rather, they are signs, symptoms, and sometimes complications that occur because our society and culture defines and dictates ones' identity.

In healthcare, we often use the words "sign," "symptom," and "complication" so it's important to take a moment to define those here.

Merriam-Webster's medical dictionary defines:

Sign as "an objective evidence of disease especially as observed and interpreted by the physician rather than by the patient or lay observer."[10]

Symptom refers to "subjective evidence of disease or physical disturbance observed by the patient."[11]

Complication refers to "a secondary disease or condition that develops in the course of a primary disease or condition and arises either as a result of it or from independent causes."[12]

---

[10]Sign. (n.d.). Retrieved March 15, 2017, from https://www.merriam-webster.com/dictionary/sign#medicalDictionary

[11]Symptom. (n.d.). Retrieved March 15, 2017, from https://www.merriam-webster.com/dictionary/symptom#medicalDictionary

[12]Complication. (n.d.). Retrieved March 15, 2017, from https://www.merriam-webster.com/dictionary/complication#medicalDictionary

An example to consider is diabetes. A "sign" would be frequent urination or increased thirst, whereas a "symptom" would be frequent infections and slow wound healing. Complications that occur over a longer period of time may be from kidney failure (which can lead to the need for dialysis), heart disease, and limb amputation.

If your doctor talks to you early about how diabetes could affect you or your loved one and the long-term complications that can arise from note merely being a diabetic, but rather from not checking your blood sugar levels, eating a poor diet full of sugar and carbs, and not taking your insulin, you may be more likely to have a better quality of life.

If you have health insurance, you are more likely to have access to professionals who teach you about the risks, nutrition, medication, and the need for preventative care, and you are provided resources to ensure you are less likely to develop long-term complications.

But, if you don't have access to education, health insurance, or professionals who understand diabetes, you become that much more likely to develop symptoms of frequent infections, weight loss, vision loss, and wounds that take longer to heal.

Now, on the other hand, if you have health insurance, you are more likely to have access to professionals who teach you about the risks, nutrition, medication, and the need for preventive care, and you are provided resources readily available to not only you, but also your spouse and your family, and you are infinitely less likely to have long-term complications.

In fact, our society and culture view the risk for developing diabetic complications as *so* important that there is representation from television characters and educational resources in all formats of media.

We hear the information every day, receive the insight provided as it applies to us individually, and it's there for recall when it directly affects us, even years down the line.

Just because our society and culture explain the existence of diabetes doesn't mean that we each become a diabetic.

Diabetes is either identified when you are a child or later in life.

For those of you who were identified as a diabetic as a child, it was imperative that the adults around you provided you with the tools you would need in both the short-term daily living, and in the long-term, to prevent complications of having amputations, becoming blind, or becoming dependent on dialysis.

If you or someone you know or love is a diabetic, you may already know some or all of this. If you are not personally a diabetic and don't understand the impact of having to check your blood sugar before each meal to see if you need insulin, that doesn't mean the signs, symptoms, and complications don't exist.

And maybe, on some level, you have care and compassion for those with "diabetic" as part of their identity.

Even if you don't have a medical degree, chances are either you or someone you care about is (or was) diabetic.

Guess what?

Chances are either you, or someone you care about is (or was) LGBTQ.

According to current research from Gallup, 4.1% of Americans self-identify as LGBTQ, which is up from 3.5% in 2012. And, a full 87% of Americans have a family member, friend, or co-worker who is lesbian, gay, or bisexual.[13] According to the Pew

---

[13]Gallup, I. (2017, January 11). In US, More Adults Identifying as LGBT. Retrieved April 18, 2017, from http://www.gallup.com/poll/201731/lgbt-identification-rises.aspx?g_source=Social Issues&g_medium=newsfeed&g_campaign=tiles

Research Center, 38% of Americans have a family member, friend, or co-worker who identifies as transgender. The number of Millennials identifying as LGBT is up from 5.8% in 2012 to 7.3% in 2016. The number of Americans owning their LGBTQ identity rose by 1.75 million people in 2012 to bring the total estimated number of Americans to 10 million LGBTQ individuals.[14]

What I am getting at here is that there are many symptoms (alcohol, drugs use, risky sex behaviors, homelessness, mental illness, or lack of education, etc.) that are not exclusive to being LGBTQ, but are often inaccurately correlated. We, as a society, continually place people in boxes, categories, or closets that we are comfortable with instead of inquiring as to what category that individual is comfortable with (if any).

We, as a society, continually place people in boxes, categories, or closets that we are comfortable with instead of inquiring as to what category that individual is comfortable with (if any).

That's worth repeating.

What I am getting at here is that there are many symptoms (alcohol, drugs use, risky sex behaviors, homelessness, mental illness, or lack of education, etc.) that are not exclusive to being LGBTQ, but are often inaccurately correlated. We, as a society, continually place people in boxes, categories, or closets that we

---

[14]Mitchell, T. (2016, September 28). 5. Vast majority of Americans know someone who is gay, fewer know someone who is transgender. Retrieved April 18, 2017, from http://www.pewforum.org/2016/09/28/5-vast-majority-of-americans-know-someone-who-is-gay-fewer-know-someone-who-is-transgender/

are comfortable with instead of inquiring as to what category that individual is comfortable with (if any).

The descriptive terms presently used to define perceived behaviors by people who identify as LGBTQ are not indicators of being LGBTQ, but rather symptoms and complications of the inability to cope with our society's expectation and projection of the only two accepted gender roles and identities (heterosexual male and heterosexual female).

When I think back to the years I spent educating physicians, case managers, social workers, patients, and families about the benefits of hospice; I remember even physicians asking me how I could be so comfortable with the sensitive topic of death and dying.

The answer was so simple. If I respect and value each and every human life, and if I have the knowledge and insight to make that journey less painful, then I need to be respectful enough to open the conversation and start a dialogue. This was so true of the healthcare professionals who, more times than not, would let a patient or family know I would be contacting them but never really say why.

If I respect and value each and every human life, and if I have the knowledge and insight to make that journey less painful, then I need to be respectful enough to open the conversation and start a dialogue.

At first, I was disheartened that they left it up to me to start the conversation, often being the first to tell them there was a life-limiting illness and that they or their loved one was going to die. And then I came to realize that they wanted their patient and family to have the information about their available choices. I also came to realize that they knew they had their own personal barriers to effectively having that conversation.

What I first thought was lack of respect was, in reality, the best they were able to offer—a resource.

And I felt humbled to be trusted with the lives they cared for.

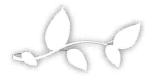

Identity and Gender Roles

"When a child is punished for their honesty, they begin to lie."

—Unknown

I'm reminded of the changes Target made in August of 2015, "We never want guests or their families to feel frustrated or limited by the way things are presented. Over the past year, guests have raised important questions about a handful of signs in our stores that offer product suggestions based on gender." Target went on to say, "Right now, our teams are working across the store to identify areas where we can phase out gender-based signage to help strike a better balance. For example, in the kids' Bedding area, signs will no longer feature suggestions for boys or girls, just kids. In the Toys aisles, we'll also remove reference to gender, including the use of pink, blue, yellow, or green paper on the back walls of our shelves."[15]

Make no mistake, as I sit here writing this, I'm remembering how I was chastised by my family for buying our grandchildren

---

[15]"What's in Store: Moving Away from Gender-Based Signs." Target Corporate, corporate.target.com/article/2015/08/gender-based-signs-corporate. Accessed 18 Apr. 2017.

pink and blue gifts for their Easter baskets. In my conscious thoughts, I have no desire to maintain that my granddaughter should wear pink and my grandson should wear blue. And yet, my subconscious conditioned or learned behavior projects the very rigid roles I know are unhealthy.

Socially and culturally, we are moving further away from strictly male- and female-identified roles. And that's a great start that will hopefully have a more positive impact on the children of our future.

But just changing the clothing options available doesn't stop the symptoms and long-term complications we set in motion at least from infancy, if not from pregnancy forward.

More than 22 different government, health, non-profit, business, and community organizations have been working together for more than 30 years to improve the health of all Americans. That group forms the Healthy People Initiative, which is governed by the Centers for Disease Control. It's more likely you've heard them referred to as the CDC.

They do that by increasing the span of healthy life, reducing health disparities, and increasing access to preventative services. To help meet these overarching goals, the CDC identified more than 300 national objectives addressing a broad array of health issues "that affect groups of people at highest risk for those areas of particular focus."[16] In any given decade, the focus may be on infants, children, teenagers, or seniors (and no, I don't mean high school).

In the past, this very process has increased awareness about Sudden Infant Death Syndrome (SIDS), hearth disease, stroke, diabetes, HIV, and cancer.

---

[16]Disparities. (n.d.). Retrieved March 15, 2017, from https://www.healthy-people.gov/2020/about/foundation-health-measures/Disparities

Change is created when health outcomes improve as a result of better healthcare.

That takes research at a clinical level.

The research is only beneficial when people have the ability to be honest without fear of discrimination.

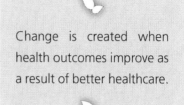

Change is created when health outcomes improve as a result of better healthcare.

Once the research is there, the information obtained then needs to be shared with professionals who can share it with society as a whole. Under the present system and process, we have spent more than 30 years acknowledging and learning about the LGBTQ community. That knowledge has not effectively trickled down to the parents and families of children who are forming their identities today, at the present moment. The knowledge that has been gained thus far is buried and not readily available to the very people it pertains to or the people who can touch the most lives with that information, unless you know what to look for and where.

By gaining better insight to special population groups at high risk of health issues, Healthy People Initiatives can set specific targets to narrow the gap between the total population and those groups with higher than average rates of death, disease, and disability.

The inclusion of those within the LGTBQ community back in the 1990s increased awareness regarding evidence-based research about the transmission of HIV, which was initially thought to only affect gay men. Fast forward to our present knowledge of transmission, testing, and treatment, which has a completely different landscape and impact today. HIV is no longer considered a terminal disease, but instead a chronic disease.

So why does that matter? The Healthy People 2010 Initiative "highlighted the need for more research to document, understand, and address the environmental factors that contribute to health disparities in the LGBT community."[17] It further identified that societal stigma and discrimination lead to inequalities in healthcare affecting LGBTQ people across the lifespan.

Although the target date was 2010, the goal was actually set back in 1997, nearly 13 years earlier.

Healthy People 2020 has sought to increase research to understand the disparities more fully (that goal was set back in 2007). The outcome of the initial research has indicated that each subgroup within the LGBTQ community experiences increased rates of common health issues. As conversation becomes more common, awareness is increased and stigma begins to decrease.

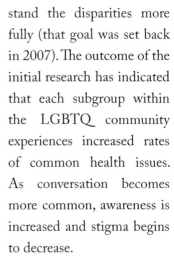

How many years and generations will it take to see a positive impact on the children being born today? What happens to the children who were born yesterday, last week, last month, last year, 10 years ago?

How many years and generations will it take to see a positive impact on the children being born today? What happens to the children who were born yesterday, last week, last month, last year, 10 years ago?

[17]Lesbian, Gay, Bisexual, and Transgender Health. (n.d.). Retrieved April 18, 2017, from https://www.healthypeople.gov/2020/topics-objectives/topic/lesbian-gay-bisexual-and-transgender-health

If conversations that teach parents about the impact of identity never happen, they don't have what healthcare professionals call "informed consent." If we don't share our knowledge and experiences, people won't know what they don't know.

The preventative information is not trickling down to the very folks who live it on a daily basis—not nearly fast enough or pervasive enough to have a positive impact for years, if not generations to come. The CDC has been diligent in urging more research for the LGBTQ community, yet the average period of time in medical school spent on teaching our present medical students about the topic is 5 hours during all of their years of residency. The nursing profession spends an average of 2.5 hours on the topic. That means the rest of the physicians and nurses who are already in practice may eventually learn through continuing education *only* if they select this specific topic. There are no current continuing education requirements for many professions regarding those within the LGBTQ community, including healthcare professionals. Just taking in to account the healthcare profession, physicians are not required to obtain any continuing education credits regarding those within the LGBTQ community, and for that matter, neither are nurses. That exists not just in my state, but in every state across the country. The licensing entities that test healthcare providers do not mandate a set curriculum or a minimum number of hours for training, nor do the policy makers who set the standards of care for all patients. One such example is a mandate that was issued following the 9/11 World Trade Center event. Since that time, all healthcare providers have been required to have *at least a* 4-hour minimum course on terrorism.

And what's worse is that our present-day youth, as well as their adult counterparts, their families, friends, and caregivers continue to experience the symptoms and complications that occur as a result of our current system of valuing personal identity and its impact.

What does any of that have to do with children? Two things for sure:

1. If you consider the example of diabetes, you'll recall we started talking about the importance of making healthy food choices for very young children. And when they were too young to manage their own food choices, we began to teach people in professions that impact children and those who care for them about healthy food choices.

2. As you consider the stages of development for children, you begin to gain insight into how society and culture dictate the male/female gender and identity roles and how that can impact the physical and emotional health of children starting as young as the age of 3.

The last three Healthy People Initiatives have included the LGBTQ community—that's three decades to make the change that we've seen so far.

And we have far to go. That means we can't sit back and rely on the CDC to do all the work. We need to work together collectively to change the impact of identity.

> We need to work together collectively to change the impact of identity.

As parents and as professionals in virtually every profession, we have unknowingly projected identity roles that are rigid in nature.

Lead Researcher and Deputy Director for the University of Warwick's Center for the Study of Women and Gender, Maria do Mar Pereira, stated in an interview with Think-Progress that, "Usually we think of gender as natural and biological, but it's not. We actually construct it in ways that have problematic and largely unacknowledged health risks." She went on to state that, "There are very strong pressures in society that dictate what is a proper man and a proper woman" and "Young people try to adapt their behavior according to these pressures to fit into society."[18]

As parents and as professionals in virtually every profession, we have unknowingly projected identity roles that are rigid in nature.

We further perpetuate those roles by asking children how they view themselves when we ask questions like, "What do you want to be the you grow up? Police officer, doctor, lawyer, teacher, nurse?" We open the dialogue for them to explore their sense of self according to the roles we have defined based on their physical male or female parts that are present at the time of their birth and we cultivate and encourage the perception of what identity they have in life, as long as it meets our needs, of course.

Picture the *"Love Is ...."* comic strip from the 1960s by cartoonist Kim Casali. I can just visualize the characters standing face to face peering in to their pants; possibly pondering the difference.

---

[18]Forcing Kids To Stick To Gender Roles Can Actually Be Harmful To Their Health. (n.d.). Retrieved April 20, 2017, from https://thinkprogress.org/forcing-kids-to-stick-to-gender-roles-can-actually-be-harmful-to-their-health-34aef42199f2

The long-term physical and mental health issues surrounding gender identity and roles are so pervasive that the American Academy of Pediatrics provides resources for pediatricians, healthcare professionals, and families about the topic. The concerning piece of news to go along with that is that, in more than 30 years of raising children, never has a pediatrician ever even approached the topic of the potential for one of my children to be something other than heterosexual. And it's not just my pediatricians over the years, I've had the same conversations with multiple parents from across the country. But it's not the pediatricians' fault, there is currently no mandatory ongoing education for practitioners.

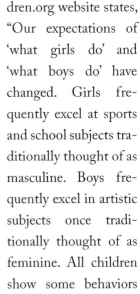

"When a child's interests and abilities are different from what society expects, he or she is often subjected to discrimination and bullying. It is natural for parents to want their child to be accepted socially. However, children need to feel comfortable with and good about themselves."

The HealthyChildren.org website states, "Our expectations of 'what girls do' and 'what boys do' have changed. Girls frequently excel at sports and school subjects traditionally thought of as masculine. Boys frequently excel in artistic subjects once traditionally thought of as feminine. All children show some behaviors that were once thought of as typical for the opposite gender—no one shows exclusively male or female traits—and this is normal."[19]

---

[19]Gender Identity Development in Children. (n.d.). Retrieved April 17, 2017, from https://www.healthychildren.org/English/ages-stages/gradeschool/Pages/Gender-Identity-and-Gender-Confusion-In-Children.aspx

HealthyChildren.org goes on to state, "When a child's interests and abilities are different from what society expects, he or she is often subjected to discrimination and bullying. It is natural for parents to want their child to be accepted socially. However, children need to feel comfortable with and good about themselves."[20]

It remains to be seen what the Healthy People 2030 goals and objectives will be and how they will be accomplished. What I do know is that another 13 years will pass before we see the full *Identity Impact.*

---

[20]Gender Identity Development in Children. (n.d.). Retrieved April 17, 2017, from https://www.healthychildren.org/English/ages-stages/gradeschool/Pages/Gender-Identity-and-Gender-Confusion-In-Children.aspx

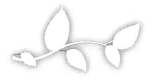

Stages of Development
and their Impact

"It's not about what it is, it's about what it can become."

—Dr. Seuss, The Lorax

What do developmental theories have to do with identity?

Everything and nothing all at once.

What I mean is that we all know that certain psychosocial theorists exist, such as Sigmund Freud, Jean Piaget, Erik Erikson, B.F. Skinner, Albert Bandura, Carl Rogers, William James, Ivan Pavlov, Lev Vygotsky, and Mary Ainsworth. Of course, some stand out in our minds more than others. And yet, sure as you recognize several of those names, there are other names you will probably not be familiar with. That's because those theorists have focused on gaining a greater insight into the LGBTQ community and have not been as visible to society in general.

Psychologists and therapists, as well as physicians and nurses, learn about theories of development, yet there is currently no uniform method of including education about gender roles and identity from birth through adulthood. There remains a lack of conversation about how identities form, when they form, and what happens to an LGBTQ person when they don't conform.

Who is teaching parents about the potential fall out when their child doesn't fit neatly into the box they and society, want to place children in?

> Who is teaching parents about the potential fall out when their child doesn't fit neatly into the box they and society, want to place children in?

Even if a physician does know the conversation needs to take place, that does not mean they know how and when to open the conversation with parents about identity formation, much less how to navigate the reality that identity forms between the ages of 3 and 5 and is set by age 7.

That occurs partly because the information is so very new and partly because they, too, have been raised with the same rigid views of gender roles and identity and they themselves may be uncomfortable.

That concept is so simple to me. Remember we talked about the roots and rings of your tree? Well, those other trees in the landscape may have different roots and rings than yours. And yet, we all help the other grow.

My hope is that by providing some awareness that these theories exist, you can at least begin to see how what we know about the emotional and psychological development of children is impacted by our overall views about gender roles and identity and how that further impacts the internal struggle with how people view themselves.

Only then, can you begin to see the potential impact on the individual who eventually identifies as LGBTQ and maybe even the impact on those afraid to own their identity.

From a clinical standpoint, whether from the perspective of a psychologist, psychiatrist, physician, nurse, social worker, therapist, or teacher, one can spend an entire career understanding and negotiating the subtle nuances among the numerous theorists and their respective pros and cons. And yet, sure as you're reading this, you are becoming aware (many of you for the

My hope is that by providing some awareness that these theories exist, you can at least begin to see how what we know about the emotional and psychological development of children is impacted by our overall views about gender roles and identity and how that further impacts the internal struggle with how people view themselves.

first time) that there are theorists who have developed an insight into the processes that those who have come to own their personal identity as a member of the LGBTQ community experience.

Not sure you see a connection? Let me help you:

Ever heard of Charlie Sheen?

"Of course!" you say? Who hasn't right?

How about the "Charlie Sheen Effect?" Ever heard of that? No?

That's because no one told you it exists.

According to the *Journal of the American Medical Association*, "On the day Sheen disclosed his HIV status there was a 265%

increase in new mentions about HIV online and more than 6,500 stories on Google News. That means that the month he disclosed his diagnosis ranked as the top 1% of HIV-related media months in 7 years.[21]

There were more than 2.75 million more searches including the term HIV including information about symptoms, testing, and condoms for prevention, and 1.25 million searches were directly related to public health outcomes."[22]

The effect of Charlie Sheen's visibility increased awareness and a search for more knowledge and information. That's impact.

Consider a different side of the same coin, so to say.

One of the reasons research is slow and challenging is because survey responders (people) are afraid to self-disclose their identity due to fear of stigma and being "outed" by others.

Even one of the most recent episodes of *Survivor*, which aired in April 2017, shows both the reality and the fear of being "outed." With increased acceptance and visibility of those who chose to live "out" as well as ally support, there are still many people in various stages of accepting their own identity who are not yet ready due to familial, societal, and religious situations.

My point is that the media has the potential to help neutralize these negative responses while simultaneously increasing general public interest and providing a means of education based on an individual's desire to learn (regardless of LGTBQ affiliation).

---

[21]MA, J. W. (2016, April 01). News and Internet Searches About HIV After Celebrity Disclosure. Retrieved February 28, 2017, from http://jamanetwork. com/journals/jamainternalmedicine/fullarticle/2495274

[22]MA, J. W. (2016, April 01). News and Internet Searches About HIV After Celebrity Disclosure. Retrieved February 28, 2017, from http://jamanetwork. com/journals/jamainternalmedicine/fullarticle/2495274

The other aspect I urge you to keep in mind is the dual reality that is experienced when society dictates your gender identity and role to be definitively male or female based on cultural expectations—while at the same time your personal identity is incongruent with what society tells you to think and feel.

For those of you who have not lived that experience, I share with you the story of when my wife (Dom) and I first met. She was in her mid-20s with naturally long, curly hair most women would pay hundreds of dollars for. She dressed the way she was expected to dress in any given situation (at work she wore suits, very often wore a dress or skirt of some kind, and when she went out, she was dressed to kill in very feminine cuts and designs). If you were to observe her walk and body posture, it was easy to see that she was almost uncomfortable in her own skin. As she began to own her identity, as she defined it for herself, she began to choose a very different style of clothing. She ultimately cut her hair (shorter and shorter, straighter and straighter). Today, although she may be dressed to kill, she no longer wears feminine cuts and designs, she choses instead to wear men's cut slacks and tailored button down shirts with a t-shirt underneath. And today, if you observed her walk and body posture, you would no longer see a dual reality or discomfort in her own skin. Instead, you would see the sure footed, confident woman who knows who she is, who she loves, and who loves her.

That, my friend, is *Identity Impact.*

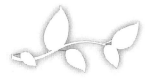

The Education of Parents and Caregivers

"I have a dream that my four little children will live one day in a nation where they will not be judged by the color of their skin, but by the content of their character."

—Martin Luther King, Jr.

I don't know about you, but on more than one occasion, I've been known to complain about the reality that children don't come with instruction manuals.

If you're of a technical nature, even when you do read the damn instructions, for some reason there are always extra parts you have no idea what to do with.

If you're like me, you might have saved those extra pieces in a little baggie in the tool box "just in case."

Developmental theories *are* the "just in case" parts that were put away in that little baggie in case you need to fix what's falling apart later on.

At some point, many of us find ourselves sitting on a therapist's sofa trying to reconfigure how we got to where we are today and why we got here. Make no mistake, we all pay a high price for that, whether it's emotional, physical, or financial. Or all of the above.

As a society, we're a little more than one loose screw and it's the not the part you think it is!

The goal is to create an awareness of several theorists whose studies impact our societal culture today and how that very culture not only has the potential to have a negative impact, but very often it *does*.

I remember when I was in high school. I went to a conservative all-girls Catholic high school on the east coast. We had a particular religion and philosophy teacher named Father Orth, who used to say, "There are no bad people in this world, just good people who make bad choices." I vividly remember sitting there in class and struggling with the incongruence back then. I was acutely aware of adults in same-sex relationships, who I perceived to be lovingly and unconditionally committed to each other (which is what I was taught existed in a heterosexual marriage). The heterosexual relationships that I personally observed from my parents and my friends' parents seemed to be different. What made those relationships more acceptable than same-sex relationships?

There was a noted incongruence between what I was taught and what I observed.

You see, I grew up in the late 70s and early 80s. Most of my friends' parents were clearly having marital issues; some were alcoholics, some were addicted to drugs. I'm sure these years resonate with many of you.

I remember my dad having friends who were same-sex couples and never having defined or even suggested anything about those relationships. In fact, I remember being intrigued by one couple in particular, not for any reason other than the compassion and understanding I silently observed occur between them. In my own case, it would be almost 23 years before that experience would resurface in my mind's eye. It would be another 2 years before I would completely understand the impact that observation had years before on my own identity.

No, I am *not* saying that having observed a lesbian couple together when I was 12 years old made me identify as a lesbian. I am indeed saying that I had no frame of reference to understand that I could be something other than a heterosexual female.

Had my parents had the insight when I was 3 to 5 years old that a normal stage of development is figuring out your identity and role in society, they may have been able to help me understand that my intrigue was a normal facet of curiosity and that there are many types of identities, roles, and loves in life. And, more importantly, they would have made it clear that whatever identity, role, and love I found in my life would have been met with acceptance, support, and unconditional love.

Years later, as I sat on a therapist's sofa, paying a lot of money to figure out that part of my identity, I remember how I described my thoughts about women. The word I chose was "intrigue." That intrigue didn't start as an adult. In fact, in retrospect, I can trace it back to the age of 5, except at that age, I didn't realize there were other options for my sense of self and for my identity.

Fast forward to this morning when I received a text from an old high school friend. Her son is about the same age I was when I first observed that lesbian couple. Today, her struggle as his parent is not that his identity is somewhere along the LGBTQ continuum but rather, how can she help guide him on his path to self discovery and acceptance while, at the same time, making sure to "keep him safe?" *She* has the foresight my parents didn't have. What she needs now are the parts from that little baggie in the tool box to help him become the best him (as he defines himself). She knows that figuring out your identity and role in society are a challenge, and now she knows she has the tools to help him. She also knows that it's okay to cry because she's scared for him, not because there is something wrong with being LGBTQ, but because she doesn't know how to make his journey easier for him. She doesn't realize that she already has. She is compassionately parenting him by allowing him the freedom to discover himself without binding him by her expectations.

I lived the "American way of life" living up to other's expectations of me. A nurturer from the age of 11 when my parents split, tending to a mother who was chronically ill, "mothering" my sister 6 years my junior, eventually becoming a young mother myself, I have continued that nurturing role to my present role in life. I married young, divorced young, married again, divorced again. All the while, I was trying to figure out why I felt like one of those hamsters on that silly wheel, going round and round and getting nowhere, fast!

I went to college right out of high school for business (the first in my family to attain a college degree) and ultimately followed in my father's footsteps in insurance sales. I went back to college again 10 years later for another degree, this time in nursing because I had taken care of my mother and her mother and was told by another adult in my life at the time that nursing was a "good profession" (not that it isn't).

All the while, I was told both verbally and nonverbally who I was and what my role in life was, based on what was expected according to our faith, our culture of origin, the culture of the region we lived in, and the culture of the generation we lived in (my roots and my climate if you get the picture).

I was raised on the east coast in the suburbs of Philadelphia. My mother had been raised in Northeast Philadelphia and was of Irish and German decent. Her family was Roman Catholic. My father was initially raised in Newark, N.J. and then in the suburbs of Philadelphia where he met my mother. He is Sicilian, his father having been an immigrant. They, too, were Roman Catholic.

I was born in late 60s and went to Catholic school until college. I was raised with the mindset of "sempre famiglia" (forever family), Sunday family dinners, and to exceed the success of my parents before me. I was also taught that Sicilian daughters become Sicilian mothers.

We may have moved 3,000 miles from where I grew up, more years than I care to count have passed, and I too, have raised my children with more than a few of the verbal and nonverbal expectations of their roles in society.

Fast forward those 25 years, after trying to figure out why things didn't fit no matter how hard I tried and the insane lengths I went to in order to conform to society and be accepted, all of which were basically a series of ineffective coping.

Although there are no appropriate stereotype behaviors to expect of those of us in the LGBTQ community, there are indeed behaviors (styles of clothing, hair, nails, cars, etc.) that can be incongruent with how we feel on the inside and yet that's what we do to be accepted. It's like keeping up with the Joneses.

My wife's favorite story to tell is about the flower dresses, high heels, and acrylic nails I wore when we first met. She lovingly jokes that I was the epitome of a "mom." I then gently (okay not so gently) remind her that first, I *am* a "mom" and second, *that's* when she fell in love with me!

Anyway, the point is: many of us do things to fit in to what society expects of us.

That doesn't mean that's who we are on the inside.

Today, you wouldn't catch me in a flower dress, high heels, and acrylic nails. I'm still that girl from school who likes jeans, a loose-fitting shirt, and denim jacket in my "heartwood," but my "bark" could be a business suit, scrubs, a lab jacket, or something in-between.

Unfortunately, my mother passed while I was still married to my second husband so I have no idea what her thoughts would have been on the subject; although she did say just before her passing that "the next time around" she was "going to be a lesbian" (which makes me personally wonder if that had some impact on her own ineffective coping and life choices).

Once I did figure out who I was and who I really loved, my dad's response was, "If I had known being a lesbian would make you this happy, I would have suggested it years ago."

Hindsight is 20/20.

As my parent, I believe my dad would have wanted to ease whatever struggles I had in life.

As a parent myself, had I had the knowledge from my life's journey thus far, I would have made different choices to make my own children's journeys in life easier—not by giving or buying them more stuff, but by opening conversation and dialogue to allow them to be who they identified for themselves.

Why did I detour and share all of this with you?

Because, as a parent of four children for more than 30 years, as a pseudo parent of two additional children, as a grandmother, and as a nurse, I chose not to believe that parents knowingly and intentionally bring children into this world (or any of the plethora of ways children come into our lives) hoping to inflict hurt or pain and see them struggle or fail in life.

I chose not to believe that parents knowingly and intentionally bring children into this world (or any of the plethora of ways children come into our lives) hoping to inflict hurt or pain and see them struggle or fail in life.

I chose to believe that, just like Father Orth said back in high school, "There are no bad people in life, just good people who make bad choices."

I also choose to believe that we make those same "bad choices" because we don't have all of the information.

I've made lots of bad choices as a parent, and I assure you that every parent has made some choice or decision that they, in retrospect, regret.

And I would venture to say that, had they had 20/20 hindsight, many of those choices would have been based on the current information if it had been available at that time of impact.

Kind of like having that instruction manual at the very beginning, you know, so you don't end up with that baggie of "extra parts" that you have no clue what to do with.

As I'm sitting here writing this, I'm reminded of the "What to Expect When You're Expecting" series of books, which came way too late for when I was pregnant with my two oldest children. Had I had them 30 years ago—especially having parents who didn't discuss puberty, periods, or basic bodily functions—I would have known that what I was experiencing was normal and anticipated. I would have known that I wasn't alone.

I would have known that closely observing and being "intrigued" by certain people or types of people was not only okay, but very normal—regardless of whether they were the same sex as me, a different sex than me, or both.

And I would have had a better support system for the journey that was ahead of me.

My parents didn't intentionally omit that information; they just didn't know. They didn't know the information for themselves and their own lives, and they certainly didn't know the impact their lack of knowledge would have on my life.

That doesn't mean they didn't love me, just that they didn't see the road ahead. They didn't have Google Maps, Siri, Waze or any other sense of direction for journey, let alone awareness of the potholes, accidents, construction, flat tires, and tickets that could lie ahead or the benefit of a having a second set path or detour that could be shorter and less harrowing with fewer potholes, accidents, flat tires, and tickets—and maybe, just maybe, have incredible scenes along the way.

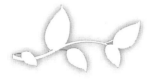

Developmental Theories 101

"Be who you are and say what you feel because those who mind don't matter and those who matter don't mind."

—Dr. Seuss

I f you're reading this and you completely recall the major developmental theorists we studied in high school and college, totally skip this section. Do not pass "Go" and do not collect $200.

If you've never learned about developmental theorists or remember that they exist but never really thought you'd actually have to use what you learned, much less ponder their impact on your everyday life, (much like my own dismay in terms of hating algebra and the unfortunate reality that not only do we have to use it every day for shopping, cooking etc., but as a nurse, I have to use it every single day, all day long, to make sure I medicate you with the right dose of prescribed medication) then this is a great crash course!

Remember in math we learned "the whole is equal to the sum of its parts?" This is exactly where that phrase comes back in to play.

The basic value of developmental theories comes in understanding how outside influences can have a positive or negative impact on our daily lives. Let's go back to that tree you drew earlier. We start with our basic roots, but depending on the basic physical needs of water, food, shelter, and warmth and the climate around us, we can grow with either positive or negative influences.

> The basic value of developmental theories comes in understanding how outside influences can have a positive or negative impact on our daily lives.

One of the interesting pieces of insight I've gained is that each theorist's information was undoubtedly presented to us based either in general format or as it would apply to whatever major we studied in school.

The missing link is that no one ever pulled all of it together in a nice, neat package that made any sense and told us what to do with that information. No one told us that our adult roles in life would impact the roots and growth of others. We become the leaves and branches on other people's trees and many of us become the rays on that sun (the climate and element that impact the growth of that next root and sapling).

We each learned the theories as they applied to our individual professions.

No one pointed out the fact that multiple professions refer to the same information from their own perspective, while having a simultaneous impact, yet we do. And when we send conflicting information and messages, we foster more conflict, confusion, isolation, guilt, and shame.

What? I'll circle back to this thought. The goal of this section is not to cover every subtle nuance between each and every theorist ... if that were the case, this would be a psychology textbook. And it's not.

The goal is, however, to remind you of some of the basics, to increase your awareness that there are other schools of thought and insight in terms of one's identity as being within the LGBTQ community, and to cultivate

We become the leaves and branches on other people's trees and many of us become the rays on that sun (the climate and element that impact the growth of that next root and sapling.)

conversation about that intersection where the impact of our societal norms and expectations (our root and our climate) have the potential to either cause a collision of epic proportions or to create an incredible scenic journey.

Maslow:

Malsow in a "nutshell" (no pun intended!)

Way back in 1943, the *Theory of Self-Actualization* was developed by Abraham Maslow. Maslow asserted that self-actualization is the growth of one's self toward fulfillment of the highest needs. The "highest need" he was referring to was the meaning of life. In his paper entitled: "*A Theory of Human Motivation,*" he theorized that human beings are motivated by unsatisfied needs, and that certain lower needs must to be satisfied before higher needs can be met and attained. Maslow used a triangle as the base for his diagram to explain each need attained. At the base of the triangle lies the most basic necessity for breathing, food, water, sexual intimacy, sleep, homeostasis, and excretion (you know, what you do in the bathroom). Wait a minute, if he included "sexual intimacy" as a basic physical need that means that each and every person has that need! I may be rocking more than a few boats with that realization, and yes, that's my goal! One's need for sexual intimacy is a basic need. These are the physiological needs we all have (the things we need physically to survive). The next level in the triangle represented the need for safety and are more psychological in nature. They include security of body, employment, resources, morality, family, health, and property. The third level is the need for love and belonging. The love referred to here is in terms of nonsexual love, the kind we refer to when we're accepted as part of a group including friends, peers, and family. Being accepted by one does not negate the need to be accepted by the other.[23]

What I mean when I say that is, although being loved and accepted by a group peers or friends is important, it does not replace the need for acceptance and love of our family of origin (whether biological or not). The fourth level is self-esteem. This section refers to respect of and by others, confidence, and achievement. Once self-esteem is attained, we are then able to set our goals to achieve self-actualization. At that final level, we become all that we can

Although being loved and accepted by a group peers or friends is important, it does not replace the need for acceptance and love of our family of origin (whether biological or not).

[23]A Theory of Human Motivation—Abraham H Maslow—Psychological Review Vol 50 No 4 July 1943.pdf. (n.d.). Retrieved February 15, 2017, from https://docs.google.com/file/d/0B-5-JeCa2Z7hNjZlNDNhOTEtMWNkYi00Y mFhLWI3YjUtMDEyMDJkZDExNWRm/edit

become. It is at this stage that we seek knowledge and peace. This is where we contemplate the meaning of life including problem solving, acceptance of facts, and lack of prejudice.

Maslow's Hiearchy of Needs

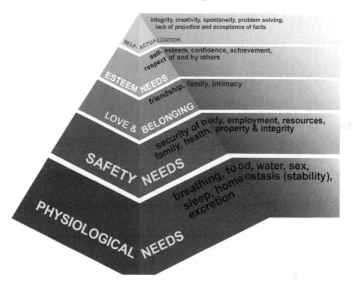

Erikson:

Another theorist whose studies are prevalent today is Erik Erikson. He first proposed his psychoanalytical Theory of Psychosocial Development in 1959 and then again in 1963.

According to Erikson, the ego identity develops as it successfully resolves crises that are distinctly social in nature. The stages involve establishing a sense of trust in others, a sense of identity in society, and impacting the next generation in preparing for their future.

Erikson believed our ego identity (identity here refers to all the beliefs, ideals, and values that shape and guide someone's behavior) is constantly changing due to new experiences and information we acquire in our daily interactions with others.

And, as we face each new stage of development, we face a new challenge that can help further develop or hinder the development of identity.

One's identity begins to form in childhood and becomes extremely important, as you no doubt are aware, during the tumultuous times of adolescence (remember I pointed that out earlier).

Erikson believed that this process continues throughout one's life and, as we experience a particular conflict, that particular conflict serves as a turning point in our development. The conflict centers on either developing or failing to develop a psychological quality or virtue.

You see, Erikson believed that our greatest personal growth potential is during times of conflict, but so too is our potential for failure.

Let me say that again:

Erikson believed that our greatest personal growth potential is during times of conflict, but so too is our potential for failure.

Meaning, if we successfully deal with conflict, we emerge from that stage with psychological strengths that will serve us the rest of our lives. If we fail to effectively cope with the conflict, we may not develop the essential skills required for a strong sense of identity and self. That is to say that successful completion of each stage results in a healthy personality and virtues or characteristics that help us resolve

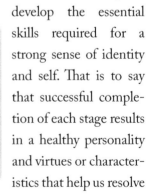

Erikson believed that our greatest personal growth potential is during times of conflict, but so too is our potential for failure.

subsequent or future crises. To complete that thought process, he also theorized that failure to complete each stage had the potential to result in decreased ability to complete further stages of development and create unhealthy personality and sense of self.

ERIKSON'S STAGES OF DEVELOPMENT

AGE	CONFLICT	VIRTUE	RELATIONSHIPS	ESSENTIAL QUESTION
Birth to 18 months	Trust vs. Mistrust	Hope	Parent	Can I trust the world?
18 months to 3 years	Autonomy vs. Shame	Will	Parent	Can I be me?
3 years to 5 years	Initiative vs. Guilt	Purpose	Family	Is it ok for me to do, move, act?
5 years to 12 years	Industry vs. Inferiority	Competence	Neighbors & School	Can I make it in the world?
12 years to 19 years	Identity vs. Confusion	Fidelity	Peers & Role Models	Who am I? Who can I be?
20 years to 25 years	Intimacy vs. Isolation	Love	Friends & Partners	Can I love?
26 years to 64 years	Generativity vs. Stagnation	Care	Household & Peers	Can I make my life count?
65 years & Over	Integrity vs. Despair	Wisdom	Mankind & My Kind	Has my life mattered?

You may want to stop and absorb what I just said for just a moment.

This is the very point of Identity Impact.

This is where we make a choice to have a positive impact on the development of a child's identity or we can continue to create rigid gender and identity roles that set our children up to fail rather than succeed.

Erikson believed that when success is experienced as a result of each basic conflict, a virtue is attained. He developed eight stages of development, some of which he felt had a greater potential for lifelong impact than others.

It's interesting to note that the ages at which Erikson identifies the greatest lifelong impact for success and/or failure are the very same ages at which our current culture and society projects a series of stereotypes on certain behaviors that our society views as negative. That means that we are effectively telling youth (and I do mean youth) at a very young age that whatever they are feeling that is incongruent with male/female gender roles is negative and unacceptable.

The easiest and most effective way I know to get through these next eight stages is to list them. Another effective way to wrap your head around it is to remember your own life or the lives of those you love as you read each stage. Each time I read the stages of development, I see yet another point of impact validated in either my own life or those I've known. If this were a text message, I'd insert the emoji with the dark hair, her eyes closed, left hand up to her face covering her forehead and eyes. Ugh. If only I knew then what I know now.

Stage 1 (ages birth to 18 months) is a time during which the conflict of Trust versus Mistrust occurs. This is where an infant looks to their primary caregiver for consistent, predictable, and reliable care. If that is experienced, the infant learns to trust that their needs will be met. This results in developing the virtue of hope. One example might be to consider an infant that is crying for hunger. When the caregiver responds by feeding the infant, the infant learns to have hope that their particular hunger cry will be responded to and their need will be met.[24]

Stage 2 (18 months to 3 years) is a time when a child begins to explore their independence. This stage is referred to as Autonomy versus Shame. This is when a child learns (hopefully in a safe environment) to make choices like what to wear, what to eat, and

---

[24]Sokol, Justin T. (2009). "Identity Development roughout the Lifetime: An Examination of Eriksonian Theory," Graduate Journal of Counseling Psychology: Vol. 1: Iss. 2, Article 14.

what to play with. It is imperative that parents allow their children to explore limits inside of an encouraging environment that is tolerant of failure. When I reflect on this development stage in my own children, I'm reminded of the time when our pediatrician explained to me that, although it was wonderful the children could make their own bed, it was important that I not remake the bed the way I wanted it made, but rather praise them for their success at independently performing the task. In everyday life, that means there's a fine balance between encouraging independence and protecting a child from failure. If children are encouraged and supported, their confidence is increased and they will be more secure in their own abilities. That autonomy results in the virtue of will. Failure to succeed results in shame.

Stage 3 (3 to 5 years) this is the Initiative versus Guilt stage. It is here that children begin to plan, initiate, and lead in games and other creative activities. When children are supported and encouraged they learn initiative. When children are criticized, ridiculed or demeaned they learn guilt. Success at this stage culminates in purpose.

So, here's where I ask: Would you rather have a strong-willed child who has the ability to go after what they want in life and feels a sense of purpose or a child who feels shame and guilt for going after what they want? Can't wrap your head around the impact of identity roles between

Would you rather have a strong-willed child who has the ability to go after what they want in life and feels a sense of purpose or a child who feels shame and guilt for going after what they want?

the ages of 3 to 5 years? Let's take gender and sex out of the equation and talk sports by using baseball, the All-American pastime.

Do you want your kid to be the one up at bat who's not afraid to hit the ball, run the bases, and get to home plate? Or are you aspiring for the child who gets nervous and strikes out at bat? Even better, do you still love and support your child when she strikes out, or do you further compound that shame and guilt because you played college ball and could have made it to the majors if it wasn't for that damn knee injury?

Here's where I secretly laugh knowing that those of you who really know me are quite impressed with my sports analogy. Wait, a lesbian who doesn't love sports? Please tell me you didn't assume all lesbians do. Because that would be a stereotype and each person's identity is so very unique.

As a side note, I should probably remind you of the research that shows this is the same age at which gender roles are formed as distinctly male or female within our current culture. That's code for: We, as a society, project gender roles onto children between the ages of 3 and 5 years old. These gender roles dictate that boys have penises, play with boy toys, grow up to marry women, and hold traditionally male occupations. Whereas girls have vaginas, play with girl toys, grow up to marry men, and hold traditionally female occupations.

Stage 4 (5 years to 12 years) is all about Industry versus Inferiority. By now, peer groups are beginning to have more impact on self-esteem and the pressure is on to win approval by displaying competencies valued by society. It's also a time when we develop a sense of pride in our accomplishments. When there is positive reinforcement, a child learns to be industrious. When there is negative reinforcement, a child learns inferiority. With appropriate balance between industry and inferiority, a child learns the virtue of competence.

Studies show two distinct pieces of information:

1) By age 7, gender roles in society are rigidly formed
2) Although the average age to "come out" is 15, a child actually begins to self-identify 5 years earlier.

That means that by 10 years old, a child is trying to sort out what they are feeling (which they may not even be able to put words to) yet knowing they need to "fit it" with their peers and the gender roles society

By age 7, gender roles in society are rigidly formed.

Although the average age to "come out" is 15, a child actually begins to self-identify 5 years earlier.

dictate. We're setting our kids up for failure.

If I were to look back at my own life, I can honestly say that when we moved to our new house when I was 5 years old, I met two sisters in the neighborhood. I vividly remember the day we met and liking both of them. I also remember studying everything about one of them in particular. I studied the way she spoke, her actions, her clothing, and her voice. I was intrigued for sure. That meeting of those two sisters took place in my neighborhood—at the intersection of Hope and Hollow. I also remember that at 5 years old, my mother dressed me in frilly dresses and I was taught to "be a lady." My best memories? Enjoying building things with my dad. I knew I was supposed to like playing with dolls and my kitchen set and yet I also liked fishing and building.

I was already being trained to see that my gender role was clearly female, yet I was drawn to study the attributes and behaviors of one of the sisters. In my later teens and early parenting years, I would come to believe that I was merely learning what other females did and was modeling myself after them when, in reality, I was very definitely attracted to one of the sisters (without being able to put a name to what I was feeling) and at the same time, was definitely wondering why in the world I didn't measure up to what I perceived was "normal."

I felt insecure and inferior. And I would feel that for many years.

Would that have been my parent's hope for me? I don't think so.

Consider in contrast Amber:

I am 11.

I'm a soccer player, friend, artist, Jersey girl, bisexual, and Jewish.

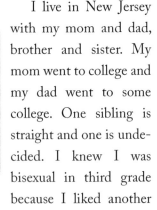

My mom has had the most positive impact on me. My friend Maggie, the one I liked, had a negative impact on me.

I live in New Jersey with my mom and dad, brother and sister. My mom went to college and my dad went to some college. One sibling is straight and one is undecided. I knew I was bisexual in third grade because I liked another girl, my best friend. I used to follow her around all the time. I don't really have any fears except if I like my close friend I might be afraid to tell them. I wanted to see how accepting friends were so

I took a survey. Some were freaked out but more said they would still be accepting and be my friend. I just did that a week or so ago. My mom has had the most positive impact on me. My friend Maggie, the one I liked, had a negative impact on me. She bullied me and put me down and I kept following her wherever she went. I started to get uncomfortable with everyone then I met another friend who helped me feel better.

Now consider Stacy, Amber's Mom:

I am 46.

I'm a Jewish, Italian, Slovak, Catholic, wife, mom, chauffeur, artist, music lover, and I am straight. I grew up in a suburb of a major east coast city. My daughter first identified as bisexual when she was in third grade and she's 11 now. She has never known that she couldn't like a girl. She was raised with acceptance of all types of diversity whether it's race, religion, or who she loved. We're Jewish so we already face bigotry, this would just be another form bullying. Being straight is easy, my fear for her is how society will treat her. I'm concerned about physical confrontation and have signed her up for self defense classes. I need to keep openly talking to her, helping to remind her to be centered

I need to keep openly talking to her, helping to remind her to be centered on who she is. I know this is going to be a hard road for her, but if you can learn those lessons when you're younger and parents can help you through it, you're better off than going through it alone when you're an adult. I hope that she has the support she needs from us and that she never questions suicide or other forms of coping.

on who she is. I know this is going to be a hard road for her, but if you can learn those lessons when you're younger and parents can help you through it, you're better off than going through it alone when you're an adult. I hope that she has the support she needs from us and that she never questions suicide or other forms of coping.[25]

Stage 5 (12 years to 19 years) is about Ego-Identity and Role Confusion. Erikson states, "The adolescent mind is essentially a mind or moratorium, a psychosocial stage between childhood and adulthood, and between the morality learned by the child, and the ethics to be developed by the adult." Erikson says that it is here where a child begins to evaluate personal values, beliefs, and goals while trying to determine their role in society. They are forming their sexual and occupational identity. Success at this stage can lead to a virtue of fidelity. Failing to establish a sense of self-identity can result in role confusion.

Are you beginning to see either yourself or someone you love having gone through these stages or the impact that unresolved conflicts at each stage can have on our development?

Consider Lisa:

I am 43 years old and I identify as a lesbian, caucasian, and atheist.

I was raised by two heterosexual parents and have one heterosexual brother. My family identifies as Catholic but were non-practicing.

I was about 11 when I first identified as lesbian. I told my friends when I was in high school but I never really had a conversation with my family about it.

---

[25]McLeod, S. (1970, January 01). Erikson's Psychosocial Stages of Development. Retrieved April 20, 2017, from https://www.simplypsychology.org/Erik-Erikson.html

How did I know? I just knew. My biggest fear was that I would be kicked out of my house, which indeed did occur. No one in my life had a positive impact, but my parents had the most negative impact. I didn't have any adults who provided support.

No one in my life had a positive impact, but my parents had the most negative impact. I didn't have any adults who provided support.

I haven't spoken to or seen my parents since 2004.

My best coping mechanism is revenge, and the greatest revenge is success. I have always strived for success and the revenge took care of itself.

My identity has made me more motivated, self sufficient, and ambitious. I knew I never had anyone to rely on, never had any support, and my family always brought me down. My identity has made me what I am today.

In contrast, consider Devon:

I am between 26 and 64 years old.

I identify as a white male, Roman Catholic of Polish Heritage.

I grew up the youngest of 10 children (seven boys, three girls) in a Philadelphia suburb, born of two blue-collar parents with a high school education. Always knowing I was gay, I came out at the age of 21 to both my family and friends. I always knew I was different, however, with the onset of puberty, I finally realized that I liked men. My biggest fear was suffocation. My father had the biggest positive impact, he was a kind man with good work ethic and taught me how to find solutions for every problem. Besides my parents, my old bosses were very inspirational and pushed me to do things that made me better. My parents were fine with my identity and handled their coping on their own. We've always spoken. Drinking has been my main coping mechanism. I have no recollection of my identity having a negative impact on my life.

Stage 6 (ages 20 to 25 years) is the stage of Intimacy versus Isolation. Successful development of intimate relationships can result in the virtue of love. Success is the development of a sense of commitment, safety, and care in a non-family relationship whereas lack of intimacy can lead to isolation, loneliness, and depression.

My father had the biggest positive impact, he was a kind man with good work ethic and taught me how to find solutions for every problem.

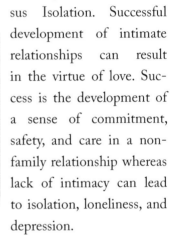

Consider Geoff:

I am 46.

I identify as a gay man, bear (grrr), democrat, business owner, son, nice guy, middle child, peacemaker, explorer, husband. Interestingly enough, for the years that I have been engaged in diversity work, I am often reminded that I am a privileged white male as the first thing that people see in me, even though that identity was not in my consciousness at all growing up. My father came from privilege, but it wasn't mine. I was taught that nothing in life comes to us for free and my family saw to it that I would endure painful reminders along the way. In fact, my grandmother felt that money was a stranglehold and a burden. I guess that is the view from the other side of a coin. Growing up I was more proud that I was born in California, that I was a Californian born in a family of early pioneers. I was from the San Gabriel Valley. Place had more importance in my identity when relating to others, just as today I am proud to be a Washingtonian from Bellevue, or when we are in Spain an American expat.

My family living situation growing up was a hot mess of drama and dysfunction moving from one situational crisis to the next. Living in the shadow of Hollywood in the LA suburbs was a foil for the notion of what is real. My parents divorced on my 6th birthday (a false indication that it was my fault, but one that I lived with). At age 6 my mother declared that I was now that man of the house, a burden I was ill prepared for. Their divorce started a war with ensuing battles that lasted for years, including 8 years of fierce custody battles. My parents made Kramer vs Kramer look like a walk in a park. In the end everyone lost. My mom was a mostly single mother trying to do her best raising three kids on a secretary's salary. We lived paycheck to paycheck; being sick or exhausted was not an option. We straddled the poverty line on every dip of the rollercoaster we were riding on. However, on the weekend, at my dad's mansion on the hill, inside the wrought iron gates on five manicured acres with a pool, stables, and tennis courts, we lived very differently. The appearance of glamour was there, but so was fear, anguish, and deep loneliness. We were never allowed to leave the property with something that my father bought for us to take home to the reality of our weekday lives. It was forbidden and made clear that choices come with consequences. My father took to the extreme that children are to be seen and not heard and my stepmother took joy in her disdain for us. We were only allowed to enter and exit the house through the servant's entrance, which made us feel less than connected to any privilege that resided in that place. We were pawns in our parents' hatred of each other, which destroyed any semblance of family or care for our individual success. I ditched a full year of high school before anyone took notice. We were essentially on our own raising ourselves. Our mother did what she could, but looked to relationships with men to dig her way out of our lows. Every year or so it seemed like a new school, place to live, and stepfather was in our lives. By the time I graduated high school I had attended 14 different schools and my mom was on husband number eight. I am sure this is more than you wanted to know, but this is what it was like.

I remember feelings from a very young age. From the age of 6 to 11 I was molested by a babysitter and his girlfriend and boyfriend, which led to a lot of identity confusion with innocence lost so early on. So I kept it to myself, with bouts of feeling confused and denial.

At about 19, I came to grips with my sexuality, but it was also the height of the AIDS crisis. So out of fear and a stronger primal pull for self-preservation, I limited my exposure to the community. At 22 I came out to most of my family as I jumped into what would be a 10-year relationship that felt secure enough to live on my own terms. After that experience ended, full acceptance and the community cheerleader mode kicked in; the activist in me was empowered.

I first knew about my identity because of the damn butter-flies in my stomach were so hard to control when anything gay was near.

My biggest fear was discovery for sure! My whole life was a string of bandages and paperclips that I held so tightly together. The conceivable fear of exposing who I was deep inside was intrin-sically tied to losing it all.

Positive and negative gets shared by my mother and father respectively. My mother's tenacity taught me strength to endure. My grandmother also had a big impact both positively and nega-tively. She loosely identified as a lesbian later in life only coming out in her 50s once her mother passed away. She was an intellectual with a thirst for knowledge and taught me to see the world with difference eyes. After coming out, people discounted her authenticity as eccentric. So her authority was always challenged and in conflict with our messy family situation. She could not be the role model she wanted to be in my life, even though she was. Her own demons and loyalty to her son (my father) ultimately destroyed our relationship.

Adults who had the most positive impact on me treated me like a person and encouraged me as a child to develop my own ideals and voice in the world. These were the adults who were out of the fray of my family's conflicts. They were in places we went to seek refuge, like our neighbor lady. We would sneak through the gate at my father's to visit her just for cookies and a game of cards. She was elderly, but it was peaceful there and we had a mutual respect and care for each other. My aunt told me when I was young not to settle into adult life until I had traveled and seen

Adults who had the most positive impact on me treated me like a person and encouraged me as a child to develop my own ideals and voice in the world.

the world. Then there's my grandmother's friend Esther (I am so very fortunate that our paths crossed). Our story is unique. We met when I was 15 and she (on my Grandmother's invitation) was living on my father's property in my treehouse. I cannot make this shit up! She was basically homeless and was introduced to me as "the artist in residence." In my treehouse! After my relationship and hers soured with my grandmother separately, she became a surrogate to me. In fact, she followed me from California to Washington and was there to support me through my coming out. We have been friends for 30+ years. Today she is 90 living in a nursing home and I am her caretaker.

I can't say how supportive my father was during my coming out as we have not seen each other since 1990 and the last time we spoke on the phone in the early 2000s (which reminded me why we don't speak). My mother of course took my gayness as her fault, since everything is about her. The first year was difficult, but she rallied in the way that she does in an over-the-top fashion. She was working for a governor at the time and arranged a civil rights conference with the keynote speaker that was a colonel. I was invited and we met, she signed her book "Serving In Silence" for me. My mother has been a community champion since then. My older sister was ashamed of me being gay. For 10 years I would visit her in Arizona and I would always have to stay at a hotel. I was never invited into her home. We have since not spoken to each other for 10 years, which is sad especially for what we went through together as kids. But time heals old wounds.

While suicide was never truly an option for me, I was pushed to my breaking point where I made the attempt in order to get the attention and help that I needed when words failed me. I was in sixth grade and made my plan known at school so that my teacher and the officials there could help me. I coped when I was young by denial. I also had what I called my "eternal hope." I knew that I could not change my current situation, but I somehow knew that when I was in control of it, it would someday get better. It was my mantra that someday things would be different and I needed patience and determination to get there. As an adult many glasses of white wine have at times helped me through when I needed to be happy and escape my problems, at least until the bottle was empty. I was never a smoker or did drugs like my sisters, but wine has always been a friend indeed. As Elaine on *Seinfeld* says, "Wine and dinner, makes a winner!"

After being fired from two jobs for being gay, I got the bump I needed to take on the challenge of becoming the entrepreneur that I had dreamed of being. Early on in life I learned that I could really only rely on myself. If my gayness was too uncomfortable for others, well then they could suck it. I knew how to survive the hard way and that is what I would do. My identity has in some regard been very freeing from the tendency to conform. Our community is not constricted from many of the rules and social norms that others have to abide by. Sure we are shunned and outcast in many ways, but in our community we can be anything we want to be. Being gay has been wonderful for me and as hard as it was to get here I would not change it even knowing that we still must fight to be ourselves. Having endured coming out makes me more courageous in other parts of my life, I am proud of that in myself. It is an achievement just to be yourself.

Stage 7 (ages 26 to 64 years) is the Generativity versus Stagnation phase. This is when we develop careers, settle into permanent relationships, and begin our own families. We're raising our own children, working within our chosen career, and involved in our community. Success leads to the virtue of care. When we fail to accomplish these goals, we become stagnant and feel unproductive and unsuccessful in life. When we've accomplished these goals, we can begin to help others generate their own success.

Consider Jersey:

I am between 26 and 64 years old.

I identify as a feminist, a woman, a lesbian, a pacifist, an Italian, and a nurse.

My parents have been married since 1968. I have an older sister and a younger brother. Yes, I am the long-suffering middle child. When I was 2 years old we moved to Iowa from California for my dad to find work as a millwright. My immediate family is really all I have ever known. I did not really ever form very many friendships as a child because my mother is not the type of person to teach us how to foster friendships. Because of this, my parents and siblings have really been my only source of support growing up.

I first started noticing girl "crushes" in the sixth grade … then I heard some girls at school making fun of someone because she "is such a lesbian " I had never heard this word before so I asked what it was. I immediately thought: Well that's what I am. But I didn't dare say anything because of the way they were making fun of this other girl. I did everything girls were "supposed to do" *I even got married!* That didn't last long. I was 25 when I stopped denying and 28 when I actually had my first lesbian "relationship."

I was 28 when I told my family and friends before I ever got involved with another woman. I think I always knew it was something that was always below the surface, and as I approached 30 I started to ask who I was living my life for and what I was hiding from. Quite honestly, my biggest fear was that I was wrong and would bring shame to the LGBT community because it really was "just a phase I was going through." It wasn't.

> My biggest fear was that I was wrong and would bring shame to the LGBT community because it really was "just a phase I was going through." It wasn't.

I always knew my family would

be supportive. They have been my most positive impact. Negative impact really became evident in the last election season, where people who I thought were supportive it turns out were not.

My mother, for sure, had the most impact. When I was growing up I had a cousin who was gay (in fact there are six of us, it runs on my Nonna's side) and my mom was always really loving and supportive of him so I knew she would be of me as well.

After I told my parents, it was a little awkward for literally about a week, but since then it's been pretty good except for the 5 years I lived with a loser and mom gave me a hard time about that. Not because she was a woman, but because she was an uneducated barely employed alcoholic I had to bail out of jail twice in 5 years.

As far as coping mechanisms that I use, I am good with me. I drink to cope with *other people*. As far identifying as LGBTQ, I am very out at work and school and if my identity has affected that, I did not really notice.

I did have a job that I was bullied out of because the nasty old bitties didn't like to see me smile when the love of my life walked in the room, but they also did that to happy heterosexuals too, so I couldn't take that personally.

Stage 8 (over 65) is the Ego Integrity versus Despair. This is when we reflect on what our life accomplishments have been. The perception of having been successful in life accomplishments leads to a sense of integrity and the virtue of wisdom whereas if we view our lives as having been unproductive and unsuccessful, we develop despair, depression, and feel a sense of hopelessness.

Before we go any further, it's important to acknowledge that homosexuality was originally classified as a mental disorder in 1968 and ultimately removed from the Diagnostic and

Statistical Manual (DSM) in 1987 (that's the year I graduated from high school to keep things in perspective). The World Health Organization (WHO) didn't remove homosexuality from its diagnosis classification until 1992 (which is one year prior to the birth of my oldest son). I would be remiss if I did not clearly address that several theories are not inclusive of the entire LGBTQ community and instead specifically addresses the "L" or Lesbian and "G" or Gay members of the community as identified back in 1979.

The Kinsey Tool:

The other piece of reference is the Kinsey Tool, developed by Drs. Alfred Kinsey, Wardell Pomeroy, and Clyde Martin, who defined the Heterosexual-Homosexual Rating Scale—more commonly known as "The Kinsey Scale." First published in *Sexual Behavior in the Human Male* (1948), the scale accounted for research findings that showed people did not fit into exclusive heterosexual or homosexual categories on either extreme side of the scale but, instead fit somewhere along the middle based on a series of thoughts, feelings, and behaviors that were not always consistent over period of time. Although many people believe this scale to be defining of sexual identity, there are actually more than 200 such tests in existence. The real value in knowing that these "tests" exist is not in the answers to sexuality that they are perceived to hold, but rather the vast sexual identities that we encounter across a continuum of time in our lives.

That means that more people are something other than strictly heterosexual than our society would have us believe. In fact, according to Gary J. Gates' April 2011 study, *How Many People Are Lesbian, Gay, Bisexual, and Transgender?*, although an estimated 3.5 % of adults (9 million) self-identified at the time (which is currently 4.5), more than 19 million American adults reported engaging in same-sex behavior and nearly 25.6 million acknowledged at least some same sex attraction. That, my friends, is more than a "minority."[26]

Consider Jordan:

I am 45 years old.

I guess I'm bi, but I'm only attracted to CIS women and trans women.

I had an ideal childhood. Lots of love, lots of laughter, lots of support. It was pretty damn great.

I was 11 years old when I realized I wanted to have sex with my neighbor friend. Sorry if that's weird, but kids have sexual urges, too.

My family and friends have always known. I knew because of my attraction.

My biggest fear I guess was in high school, it was that I'd be found out. By college, it was no big deal.

My parents have had the greatest positive impact. Great parents, great upbringing. Totally supportive.

My greatest negative impact? My first wife. She knew I was bi when we married, and she agreed to it. Then, later, she changed her mind.

The most impact was made on me by teachers, college professors, and my first editor, who showed me how to write.

No one helped my parents and I have always had a loving, completely open, and supportive relationship.

I used to drink when I was younger. Not because of parental adjurations, but because of societal mores that it was somehow "wrong." That I shouldn't want to be with trans women or boys.

---

[26]Gates, G. J. (2011, April). How many people are lesbian, gay, bisexual and transgender? Retrieved April, 2017, from https://williamsinstitute.law.ucla.edu/wp-content/uploads/Gates-How-Many-People-LGBT-Apr-2011.pdf

My identity hasn't affected my life, education, and career. I got through it. My current wife knows I'm bi, she's bi, and we have a wonderfully fulfilling relationship.

Maslow (check), Erikson (check), next theorist you ask?

Cass:

The next theorist to consider is Vivienne Cass. I would venture to say many of you have never heard of her. Cass developed the Homosexuality Identity Model back in 1979 when many within the LGBTQ community were fighting for basic human needs and civil rights. Cass theorized that there are several stages one transitions through that can be impacted by the interaction between the individual and their environment. Getting that root and climate reference again?

Cass's theory is based on two assumptions:

1) Identity is acquired through developmental processes
2) The center of stability directly relates to an interaction process that occur between an individual and their environment.

Cass also indicated that the length of time to proceed through all six stages varies from person to person. She also noted that *identity foreclosure* is possible at each stage.

Identity foreclosure refers to a person's choice to *not* develop their LGBTQ identity any further.

Case asserted that there are both private (personal) and public (social) aspects of one's identity.

According to www.learningtheories.com, Identity Foreclosure is the status in which the

Identity foreclosure refers to a person's choice to *not* develop their LGBTQ identity any further.

adolescent seems willing to commit to some relevant roles, values, or goals for the future. Adolescents in this stage have not experienced an identity crisis. They tend to conform to the expectations of others regarding their future (e.g., allowing a parent to determine a career direction).[27]

In other words, we conform to who or what we believe we should be rather than achieving our identity after we have explored ourselves and our feelings.

> We conform to who or what we believe we should be rather than achieving our identity after we have explored ourselves and our feelings.

I would venture to say more than a few of us have had this experience, whether it relates to our college, career, wedding, or spouse. Think of it like the movie *Ground Hog Day* with Bill Murray and Andie McDowell, except it is a masquerade and the mask on the outside doesn't match the person under the mask … regardless of how cool they are.

Consider Barrett:

I am 26 to 64 years old. I identify as male, black, Buddhist

I was raised in California by a two-parent working class household. I have one younger male sibling. I was a pre-teen when I first identified as LGBTQI. I was 21 years old when I told my friends and 29 years old when I told my family. I knew by instinct and my biggest fear was judgment.

---

[27]Identity Status Theory (Marcia). (2016, September 03). Retrieved March 15, 2017, from https://www.learning-theories.com/identity-status-theory-marcia.html

My mother and grandmother had the most positive impact. I don't have any examples for negative impacts other than racist people I have crossed paths with.

My mother is naturally liberal. My father and I did go over a year without speaking and we later reconciled. I don't have any particular coping mechanisms. My LGBTQ identity has affected my life, education, and career as I was in the closet for many years professionally and easily passed as straight. My career skyrocketed after coming out of the closet.

Cass identifies the six stages as follows:

1. Identity Confusion, awareness of oneself as different or other than the societal determined role.
2. Identity Comparison, a comparison of one's own feelings and emotions to those traditionally identified as heterosexual.
3. Identity Tolerance, accepting a non-heterosexual identity "I probably am ....," an awareness that there is an in-congruency between one's perceived identity and the identity indicated by societal roles.
4. Identity Acceptance, when a person acknowledges and begins to "normalize" their identity, possibly becoming more active within the LGBTQ community.
5. Identity Pride, a sense of becoming fully immersed within the LGBTQ community.
6. Identity Synthesis, full acceptance and synthesis of both LGBTQ identity with former heterosexual life. The previously viewed sense of "us" versus "them" no longer holds true.

Math Equation: 15 − 5 = 10:

If the average age a child comes out is 15 and they start to self-identify five years earlier at the age of 10, that means that they're working through Erikson's 5th stage of Ego-Identity and Role Confusion while, and possibly simultaneously, transitioning through Cass's Homosexuality Model.

Imagine if you will, the creation of the perfect storm that has the ability to create the brightest and most vivid spring season you have ever witnessed or the mass casualties from a collision at the busiest intersection. Which would you prefer?

Maslow (check), Erikson (check), Cass (check). That means D'Augelli is next:

D'Augelli:

In 1994, Anthony D'Augelli developed the Homosexual Life-Span Development Model based not on stages of development but rather a more fluid transition in and out of various stages at different times and more than one time.

It's important to note that, although D'Augelli's Homosexual Life-Span Development Model specifically addresses the lesbian, gay, and bisexual members of the larger LGBTQ community, it is not completely inclusive of all the ways people within the LGBTQ community identify as that continues to evolve. In his theory, D'Auggelli indicates that the processes identified can occur one time, multiple times, or not at all, and that there is no particular order, rather it is more of a journey during the course of one's lifespan depending on when and if one has a sense of safety in living their identity. He is attributed with introducing sexual identity as a spectrum rather than the binary (two) roles of male/female

Those stages are, in no particular order:

1. Entering a Lesbian, Gay, Bisexual Community
2. Exiting a Heterosexual Identity
3. Developing a Personal Lesbian, Gay, Bisexual Identity

4. Developing a Lesbian, Gay, Bisexual Intimacy Status
5. Claiming an Identity as a Lesbian, Gay, Bisexual Offspring (child)
6. Developing a Lesbian, Gay, Bisexual Identity

Consider Alicia:

I am between the ages of 20 to 24 years old.

I identify as a woman, trans, pansexual, white, student, Christian, and coordinator.

I grew up in a suburb of Las Vegas. Family was there when I needed them and hesitant but supporting. I grew up in a family of college graduates. We were an average family. I had difficult brothers.

I first realized I was trans when I was in sixth grade but didn't make any strides until I was a senior in high school. I came out to my parents twice—once in sixth grade, then I went into the closet again, then re-came out during my junior year of high school. I didn't come out to any of my other friends until the last day of high school.

I knew because it kinda just made sense and I always new I would one day grow up to be a woman.

My biggest fear was social acceptance.

The people that helped me the most are probably my mom, Dina Proto, my boss Katrina, and my group of friends that I met after I went to college. The hardest people were my friends back in high school because I knew they would never accept me if I came out to them.

I'm not sure who helped my parents cope, but when I was coming out they spoke with different people like my counselor, my mentor, and some people in the community. Through it all we were able to be cordial, but I only really opened up to them after I left the house because while I lived there I had to follow their rules. I also remember being afraid they might not pay for college if they didn't accept me being trans.

I mostly play video games to cope with my thoughts and feelings when I'm thinking through something. My identity gave me a community and opened me up to be an understanding person but it has not directly affected my work or career. It did force me to have difficult financial discussions and disabled me to have children, which was difficult for me to accept.

Consider in contrast Mattie:

I am between the ages of 26 and 64

I'm Italian, Catholic, a Yankee transplant living in the South and a big-time sports fan.

I grew up in Pennsylvania, but my dad was transferred to South Carolina after my sophomore year in high school. My family includes my parents and a younger sister. We were a typical middle class family. Both parents worked full-time. I had a happy childhood.

I first thought I was gay right as I was finishing college (around 21 years old) but I didn't want it to be true so I had the mentality of "I would rather be dead than gay" so there was a period of denial. Then, when I was around 25 or 26, I had an epiphany walking through the building at work that I was gay and I was completely okay with that fact—I literally said under my breath, "I am gay" as I was walking and I lit up inside being able to say it to myself.

I first knew I was gay because I developed a crush on a co-worker who I played softball with on the company team and it was like being a teenager again with that "young love" feeling about the situation.

I told my family and friends in stages, starting out with people I thought would handle it better than others and then onto those who I knew would take this information badly.

My biggest fear was being rejected by people once they found out I was gay. I haven't really had a negative experience when I have told people, in fact a few people said it wasn't really a shocker when I told them.

I can't think of any negative impacts on my relationships, but from the positive side I would say my sister, who not only was accepting, but is the only person in my family who explicitly knows my "roommate" Lisa is actually my partner of almost 15 years. My parents probably realize we are together (and one day in a pre-menopausal fit I might flat out say something) but it is never expressed verbally.

There really isn't any one adult that made a positive impact on me that I can think of, the person who I wish I could say is my Aunt who died in 2001, about 2 years after I came out. She and I were very close. I hate that she never got to meet Lisa.

My parents are an interesting situation. I knew they would have a hard time with this news. In fact, my Aunt told me to send them a letter first to break the news and then follow it up by going to their house to talk—that way I would not have to see my mom's face when she first heard the news. I told them I was gay over 15 years ago and in that time the word gay or any conversation about being gay has never happened with my mom. She is very much the ostrich—burying her head in the sand about things. My dad is a little more open about it (he likes to let me know when he hears about a celebrity coming out in case I had not heard the news yet) but there really isn't much talk.

I never drank, smoked, or used drugs but there were some suicidal thoughts in my early 20s from depression that was more than just thinking I was gay (it was only a part of it). I dealt with those feelings and overcame them and am very happy with the life I have now.

I don't think my identity has had any affect on my life, education, or career.

Maslow, Erikson, Cass, D'Augelli, check, check, check, and check

On to Bilodeau and Renn:

In "Analysis of LGBT Identity Development Models Reveals Fluidity, Complexity, and Contradictions" Bilodeau and Renn state that the "differences among the stage models illustrate the difficulty of using only one model to understand the complex psychosocial process."[28] They go on to address the reality that "few models exist that specifically address development issues of lesbian, gay, and bisexual adolescents."[29] That was written as recently as 2005. What that means is that this information is so very new to professionals that even they themselves are still learning and have yet to begin to educate the rest of society.

So far we've covered Maslow, Erikson, Cass, D'Augelli, Bilodaeu, and Renn.

Heng (final check):

In an abstract by Kenneth Heng at University of Calgary entitled, "Models That Change, the Study of Gay Identity Development" Heng states, "While the models certainly contain different themes influenced by society, we see that there are many aspects

---

[28]B, B. L., & R, K. A. (n.d.). Analysis of LGBT Identity Development Models and Implications for Practice. Retrieved February 02, 2017, from https://msu.edu/~renn./BilodeauRennNDSS.pdf

[29]B, B. L., & R, K. A. (n.d.). Analysis of LGBT Identity Development Models and Implications for Practice. Retrieved February 02, 2017, from https://msu.edu/~renn./BilodeauRennNDSS.pdf

that do not change. For instance, the feelings of difference, sensitization, and alienation are common in virtually all models. However, this may not always be the case. As society is changing to become more tolerant and accepting, and as the rate of that evolution is accelerating, the future of gay identity development models progressively becomes more uncertain. If and when stigma is removed, then the defining feature of gay identity development is also removed. It is plausible that in its place will be a general model of sexual identity development, where homosexual and heterosexual paths diverge innocently and quietly in a society that does not value one over the other."[30]

Let's bring it on home.

Remember my reference to math class? We learned that "the whole is equal to the sum of its parts?" This is exactly where that phrase comes into play. The basic value of developmental theories comes in understanding how outside influences (roots and

If and when stigma is removed, then the defining feature of gay identity development is also removed. It is plausible that in its place will be a general model of sexual identity development, where homosexual and heterosexual paths diverge innocently and quietly in a society that does not value one over the other.

---

[30]H, K. (2007, March). Models that Change: The Study of Gay Identity Development. Retrieved February 02, 2017, from https://dspace.ucalgary.ca/bitstream/1880/47539/1/Heng_2007.pdf

climate) can have a positive or negative impact on our lives on a daily basis.

This is the very point of Identity Impact.

This is exactly where we can chose to have a positive impact on the development of a child's identity or we can continue to create rigid gender and identity roles that set a child up to fail rather than succeed. How is that possible?

It's interesting to note that the ages at which Erikson identifies the greatest lifelong impact for success and/or failure (ages 5 to 18) are the very same ages at which our current culture and society project a series of stereotypes on certain behaviors.

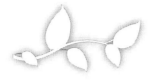

The Challenge with Stereotypes

So what's the problem with a stereotype? For those of you who remember *The Breakfast Club*, or who lived *The Breakfast Club*, you well know that there is the external that society judges us by and the internal that we all aspire to be (the "bark" versus the "heartwood"). The impact of identity and the collision of roles personified.

For those of you who don't remember the 1985 coming-of-age movie with the ever-famous "Brat Pack," it revolved around five very seemingly different teenagers from different cliques or social groups (based on stereotypes of course). They each found themselves in Saturday detention for a host of reasons. They realize through their time spent together that they are each more than their outward appearance or stereotype would have you believe. And, in fact, although their outward expression of self was different, internally, they were more alike than they had realized. It culminates in a "Kumbaya" moment where new respect and even relationships are formed.

Truth be told, I hope that, on some measure, we will come to the same space of understanding.

Although that remains to be seen.

How many of you reading this are familiar with the belief that people within the LGBTQ community often have depression, suicide ideations and attempts, substance and alcohol abuse, risky sex behaviors, breakdowns in family, and increased homelessness?

Those are stereotypes projected by society to prove that being somewhere along the LGBTQ continuum is "less than." In an article entitled "LGBT Strength: Incorporating Positive Psychology into Theory, Research, Training, and Practice," Vaughan and Rodriguez discuss the intersection of the identities possessed by those within the LGBTQ community as well as the common experiences related to rejection of traditional heterosexism norms and the stress that is encountered as a consequence. It's interesting to note that

LGBT psychology literature has all too often relied on heterosexual and cisgender reference groups as the norm with respect to psychological health, primarily framing the experiences of LGBT individuals through the lens of psychopathology. As a result, strengths that could be ascribed to the LGBT experience have been overlooked within training and practice.

although the fields of healthcare and psychology are beginning to identify the negative psychological effects of the minority stress (those healthcare disparities we talked about) that LGBTQ individuals experience. Vaughan and Rodriguez state, "LGBT psychology literature has all too often relied on heterosexual and cisgender reference groups as the norm with respect to psychological health, primarily framing the experiences of LGBT individuals through the lens of psychopathology. As a result, strengths that could be ascribed to the LGBT experience have been over-looked within training and practice. While positive psychology is actively being incorporated into clinical and counseling psychology curricula, broadening the paradigm to include LGBT individuals has generally not been included in the discussion."[31]

That means that, while we are hoping to create awareness and inclusion, we are potentially creating an unintentional bias about the meaning of sexual and/or gender minority status and how that affects not only the individual, but their family and the those around them by the very healthcare professionals who are sought out for their knowledge and skill set. This illustrates that professionals are not receiving the training required to care for those within the LGBTQ community.

While we are hoping to create awareness and inclusion, we are potentially creating an unintentional bias about the meaning of sexual and/ or gender minority status and how that affects not only the individual, but their family and the those around them by the very healthcare professionals who are sought out for their knowledge and skill set.

If you are, or have ever been, in a leadership position, undoubt-edly, you've heard the phrase: "people live up to the expectations we set for them." That theory is, unfortunately, alive and well in our current approach to people who identify along the LGBTQ

[31]Lytle, M. C., Vaughan, M. D., Rodriguez, E. M., & Shmerler, D. L. (2014, October 01). Working with LGBT Individuals: Incorporating Positive Psychology into Training and Practice. Retrieved February 15, 2017, from https://www.ncbi.nlm.nih.gov/pmc/articles/PMC4276565/

continuum. Make no mistake, the external emotional stressors of being "less than" have a lasting impact on not only the emotional but physical health of those within the LGBTQ community. We have the power to change that impact in a positive way.

What that means is, if we were to instead highlight the positive strengths of being LGBTQ, we would be encouraging a movement away from negative coping toward positive coping.

> If we were to instead highlight the positive strengths of being LGBTQ, we would be encouraging a movement away from negative coping toward positive coping.

If we go back to Erik Erikson's Stages of Development, he points out that there is a connection between stress and psychological growth and healthy development of personality traits.

What Erikson is referring to is the development of stress-related growth (SRG). When we encounter what we perceive to be a stressful situation, we have the opportunity to grow and develop healthy personality traits. That is stress-related growth. I recently had opportunity to hear Allison Levine keynote at a local conference. She served as the first American Women's Everest Expedition team captain and is *The New York Times* bestselling author of *On the Edge: Leadership Lessons from Everest and Other Extreme Environments.* Allison spoke of her courage to face adversity and the power of resilience and how that ultimately advanced her personal development of strength, wisdom and authenticity.

I have a clear understanding that I personally have been afforded a very unique vantage point. As a nurse, I have seen firsthand, the emotional and physical issues faced by the LGBTQ community. I have experienced it not only as a nurse, but also as a patient. As a business owner, my customers (both LGBTQ and their families) have shared their experiences. As a visible community leader (who happens to be a nurse) I have seen it. My wife always says I can go anywhere and people will share their story with me. I'm honored to be that safe space. I also understand that being that safe space means that I can drive positive change. I can help impact identity—yours and mine.

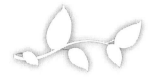

Gender Identity
and Role Formation

ere's where I put on my nursing hat and own that aspect of my identity.

Those "stereotypes" of projected behavior are not traits owned by those within the LGBTQ community but rather signs and symptoms of a larger more prolific disease. It's a poor attempt to make those who are different than we perceive ourselves as inferior. We as a society project or dictate what is "normal," even to the point that Americans go into financial debt to keep up with the Joneses instead of being happy with who we are and what we have.

My view may be somewhat skewed based on where I reside in the country—but not that skewed.

Living in Las Vegas, where gambling is a way of life for many, I'm used to seeing people in debt. As a society, we think nothing of enjoying today and opting to pay the debt tomorrow. Think about it, how many of you are living pay check to pay check or worry that you don't have enough money in the bank for a basic emergency but you have the latest and greatest tools of technology or the newest car with the latest gadgets?

How many of you lost or were in danger of losing your homes during the housing crisis of 2008?

We trade our cars in every few years, we live in houses we can't afford and buy name brand clothes so that we have the appearance that we've "made it."

When really, what appears to be so, isn't. And at some point, we need to pay that debt. We can't avoid it forever. It eventually catches up to us.

At some point, we pay a very high price for keeping up appearances to maintain societal expectations. I'm afraid that's what's happening to those within the LGBTQ community.

Remember in Erikson's Stage 3 (ages 3 to 5 years) where children are learning that children with boy "parts" play with boy toys, grow up to marry women, and hold traditionally male occupations? Children with girl "parts" play with girl toys, grow up to marry men, and hold traditionally female occupations. When we support or affirm a child's behavior according to society's projected gender roles, the children who naturally would identify as heterosexual are affirmed in their identity and learn initiative, which results in the virtue of purpose. When we negate, criticize, ridicule, or demean a child's behavior based on society's projected gender roles, the children who naturally would identify as "other than heterosexual" are negated in

At some point, we pay a very high price for keeping up appearances to maintain soci-etal expecta-tions. I'm afraid that's what's happening to those within the LGBTQ community.

their identity learn guilt, and may never achieve the virtue of purpose.

By age seven we learn that without conforming to society's expectations of our gender, we are considered "less than."

From that point through adulthood, children can ultimately learn to perceive themselves as inferior, with low self esteem, with difficulty in identifying their role in society in terms of not only relationships but professionally. This can further lead to isolation, loneliness, and depression, as well as the potential to fail in development of relationships and furtherance of career attainment. This, in turn, can lead to further feelings of despair, depression, and a sense of hopelessness.

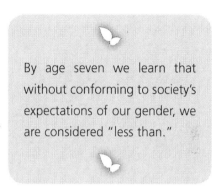

By age seven we learn that without conforming to society's expectations of our gender, we are considered "less than."

It is here that my concern as both a mother and nurse are greatest. At some point, the debt we've put off for maintaining appearances will come due.

Remember when I said I wished we got an instruction manual with kids?

This is where it would come in handy. I wish someone had taken the time to teach me (much in the same way I was taught what to expect during the "terrible twos") that my children were forming their sense of self identity from ages 3 to 5 and that by 7 years of age their sense of acceptable gender roles would be rigid. I would have wanted to know how that information could impact my children. I would have wanted to know how reinforcing the "normal" male/female gender and sex roles set an expectation for my children that they live up to society's expectations for those roles and how that could affect their mental and physical health.

And I would have wanted guidance on how to help them and how to cultivate conversations that enabled them to gain a greater understanding and acceptance of themselves (however they identified themselves versus how I or society identified them).

> I would have wanted guidance on how to help them and how to cultivate conversations that enabled them to gain a greater understanding and acceptance of themselves (however they identified themselves versus how I or society identified them).

As a parent, I have always believed that if I raised my children to be kind, smart, compassionate, and productive members of society who can provide for themselves financially and have a life they can be proud of, then I would have succeeded as a parent. That has never meant defining their religious/spiritual beliefs or their career path for them.

I did not raise my children with the mindset that they would follow in my footsteps, but rather, create their own.

The footsteps that make them proud of themselves.

And when that happens for them, I too, am proud.

That means loving them unconditionally, celebrating the things they feel make them successful, and knowing they are writing their chapters as I, too, am writing mine—even when it makes me uncomfortable or I have a different vision for them.

Make no mistake, I have definitely made mistakes—just ask any of my children!

And I have several baggies with loose parts for sure. But I can say this, I love each of my children (biological, adopted, and otherwise) for the people they are.

My hope and wish for them is that they are healthy, safe, and happy in life with as few regrets as possible.

We all have them (regrets) but they don't need to define us, rather they can guide us.

It still remains to be seen what life has in store for each of them.

I know this though, even when I don't understand their choices or they are different than mine would be for whatever reason; I love my children and nothing is worth jeopardizing their health and safety, nor our relationship—including being "overprotective," which I have been accused of on more than one occasion.

One of the interesting pieces of insight I've gained is that each theorist's information was undoubtedly presented to us as general information or as it would apply to whatever major we studied in school.

The missing link is that no one ever took the time to explain why that information was important and how it would impact my life or the lives of those I cared about.

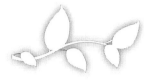

Individual and Collective
Use of Developmental Theories

It was like learning an algebra equation and having no clue what the hell I was supposed to do with it.

I know now that, if a physician orders a medication in a certain dose and the pharmacy gives me the same medication in a different dose, I need to use algebra to convert what I actually received to what was actually ordered. The impact if I don't use algebra to help me is that I can over-medicate you and you can stop breathing or die *or* I can under-medicate you, in which case you won't die, but you may write a complaint to the hospital that your pain wasn't managed. If, instead, I use the knowledge I learned in algebra, I can manage your pain, keep you breathing, and possibly receive a letter that you had a better experience than you had hoped for.

We each learned the theories either at some point in high school or in college as they applied to our individual career paths.

Whether you have a degree in medicine, education, psychology, business, marketing, media, or engineering, we all took

"Psychology 101." Yet no one ever intentionally pointed out that many professions use the same stages of development to guide their actions.

Let's look at the whole picture.

Imagine your 10-year-old self.

If I think back to the 10-year-old me, I know that I was in fifth grade with Ms. Jones. (She dated the lead singer of the J Geils Band). No judging—this was the beginning of the MTV era! Soap operas were popular as was late-night television, *Saturday Night Live*, and HBO. It was also just before our school got its first set of computers. My world of influence (and that of my parents to provide them education) was our community, our church, our school, the pediatrician, the therapists we ended up seeing because of my parents divorce, our family members, and friends. My circle of influence had the greatest impact on what I perceived was "normal."

We have no concept of how the layers of mixed or negative messaging by each profession set the stage for continued destruction of our children and ultimately our society.

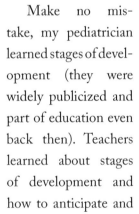

Make no mistake, my pediatrician learned stages of development (they were widely publicized and part of education even back then). Teachers learned about stages of development and how to anticipate and identify a child who was "at risk" and make a referral to therapists and/or psychologists. Media professionals learned about stages of development so they knew how to target each age group. Business majors learned about stages of development so they could develop their business models for their ideal consumer. Get the picture?

The powerful impact each has on a child's perception is mind-blowing.

Each of us ultimately refers to the same information from our own perceived perspective, while at the same time, being unaware that there is a simultaneous point of impact we all have.

To compound that, we have no concept of how the layers of mixed or negative messaging by each profession set the stage for continued destruction of our children and ultimately our society.

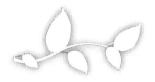

The Intersection
of Hope and Hollow

"Don't let the noise of others' opinions drown out your own inner voice."

—Steve Jobs

W hen we demand there is only one identity that is the accepted "norm" in our society based on male/female gender roles, the impact creates a collision of the struggle to succeed, as explained by Erikson's Stages of Development and Cass's or D'Augelli's Development Models.

Be mindful of the intersection between being Hollow and being full of Hope.

It's hard enough to build something without that damn instruction manual and yet, harder still when you have extra pieces that don't fit or

When we demand there is only one identity that is the accepted "norm" in our society based on male/female gender roles, the impact creates a collision of the struggle to succeed.

when what you've built falls apart. It's even harder when it falls apart beyond repair.

The hardest and most painful thing of all, is to watch a child fall apart—especially if the fall was preventable.

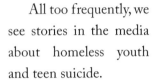

The hardest and most painful thing of all, is to watch a child fall apart—especially if the fall was preventable.

All too frequently, we see stories in the media about homeless youth and teen suicide.

All too frequently, we see stories of depression complicated by self-medication with drugs and alcohol.

According to a recent report from the CDC, "A nationally representative study of adolescents in grades 7 to 12 (ages 13 to 18 years old) found that lesbian, gay, and bisexual youth were more than twice as likely to have attempted suicide as their heterosexual peers."[32]

And according to the study, "Serving Our Youth 2015: The Needs and Experiences of Lesbian, Gay, Bisexual, Transgender, and Questioning Youth Experiencing Homelessness" by the Williams Institute of Law at UCLA, "Providers reported a median of 20% identify as gay or lesbian, 7% identify as bisexual, and 2% identify as male questioning their sexuality. In terms of gender identity, 2% identify as transgender female, 1% identify as

---

[32]Institute of Medicine (US) Committee on Lesbian, Gay, Bisexual, and Transgender Health Issues and Research Gaps and Opportunities. The Health of Lesbian, Gay, Bisexual, and Transgender People: Building a Foundation for Better Understanding. Washington (DC): National Academies Press (US); 2011. 4, Childhood/Adolescence. Available from: https://www.ncbi.nlm.nih.gov/books/NBK64808/

transgender male, and 1% identify as gender queer."[33] The study goes on to state that: "The most commonly cited reason for homelessness among LGBTQ clients, from the perspectives of agency staff, was due to being forced out by parents or running away because of their sexual orientation or gender identity/expression (i.e., SOGIE) (Figure 12). This is followed by family issues, such as substance abuse, mental illness or violence in the household, and youth being aged out of foster care systems with nowhere stable to live for both LGBQ and transgender youth. A higher proportion of respondents reported that lack of culturally competent services was a reason for homelessness among transgender youth than they did for LGBQ homeless youth."[34]

When I was 10 years old, I didn't get the chance to appropriately develop my own sense of identity. I was busy living the life my parents had created for me, in a majority of my personal roles that I would own for many years. I took my cues of who I was supposed to be, what should be important to me, what made me successful from the verbal and nonverbal messages I received from the adults influencing my life. And they did it unintentionally.

---

[33]Serving Our Youth 2015: The Needs and Experiences of Lesbian, Gay, Bisexual, Transgender, and Questioning Youth Experiencing Homelessness. (2015, June 05). Retrieved February 15, 2017, from https://williamsinstitute.law.ucla.edu/research/safe-schools-and-youth/serving-our-youth-2015-the-needs-and-experiences-of-lesbian-gay-bisexual-transgender-and-questioning-youth-experiencing-homelessness/

[34]Serving Our Youth 2015: The Needs and Experiences of Lesbian, Gay, Bisexual, Transgender, and Questioning Youth Experiencing Homelessness. (2015, June 05). Retrieved February 15, 2017, from https://williamsinstitute.law.ucla.edu/research/safe-schools-and-youth/serving-our-youth-2015-the-needs-and-experiences-of-lesbian-gay-bisexual-transgender-and-questioning-youth-experiencing-homelessness/

Until one fateful day at the age 34. In retrospect, I had *identity foreclosure* on some subconscious level, I had denied my identity as a lesbian.

When I did finally own my identity, I (along with my family) was certain I was having a mental breakdown. I know from conversations with my dad that the hardest part of that journey for him was watching me struggle emotionally with the dilemma of that dual identity. How could I have been married to a man and have children and now be a lesbian? My dad was certain it was a "college experiment." I remember, not so politely, reminding him that college had been almost 20 years earlier. I definitely had an emotional fall for more than a year. And not only did my dad watch that struggle, but so did my children. They watched their strong, independent, and successful mother question every single aspect of her life. It took me more than a minute to regain my sea-worthy legs.

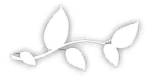

Long-Term Complications

"Let's raise children who won't have to recover from their childhoods."

—Pam Leo

Remember those "stereotypes"—the depression, suicide attempts, substance and alcohol abuse, risky sex behaviors, breakdown in family, and increased homelessness experienced by those in the LGBTQ community?

They're so much more than stereotypes.

Many people in society resort to drugs, alcohol, gambling, shopping, and sex as a means to cope with daily stressors. In an article by Jerome Hunt, "Why the Gay and Transgender Population Experiences Higher Rates of Substance Use," Hunt explains that, "The stress that comes from daily battles with discrimination and stigma is a principle driver of these higher rates of substance use, as gay and transgender people turn to tobacco, alcohol, and other substances as a way to cope with these challenges. And a lack of culturally competent healthcare services also fuels high substance use rates among gay and transgender people."[35]

---

[35]Hunt, J. (n.d.). Why the Gay and Transgender Population Experiences Higher Rates of Substance Use. Retrieved March 25, 2017, from https://www.

In fact, Hunt further brings to light that there have been instances where the LGBTQ community has been specifically marketed to. "Tobacco and alcohol companies have exploited gay and transgender social networks to aggressively market their products for decades. In the early 1990s tobacco companies surveyed gay men for branding choices, which resulted in a new program called Subculture Urban Marketing, or SCUM, which targeted minority gay men in San Francisco."[36]

Those of you reading this who are psychologists, psychiatrists, therapists, social workers, or guidance counselors already know that the "stereotypes" indicate a bigger issue at hand. And, no doubt, you are often one of the first resources parents go to when there's "something wrong" with their child. And then it's your job to figure out what the hell happened and how they ended up in your office.

By then, the child undoubtedly has been labeled with a host of diagnoses or terms, the child feels hopeless and the parent(s) feel hopeless. It may even be the case that the child is self-harming and may have even required medical treatment to some varying degree.

Let me just add to the collision at that intersection.… Did you know that those within the LGBTQ community have higher rates and complications of health issues that are further impacted by the mere fact of being LGBTQ, *not* because of the "stereotypes" that are used to define us but of the ineffective coping caused by years of trying to live up to the Joneses' way of life.

---

americanprogress.org/issues/lgbt/reports/2012/03/09/11228/why-the-gay-and-transgender-population-experiences-higher-rates-of-substance-use/

[36]Hunt, J. (n.d.). Why the Gay and Transgender Population Experiences Higher Rates of Substance Use. Retrieved March 25, 2017, from https://www.americanprogress.org/issues/lgbt/reports/2012/03/09/11228/why-the-gay-and-transgender-population-experiences-higher-rates-of-substance-use/

I'm wondering if you have any concept of the tangible health complications experienced by those of us within the LGBTQ community.

Remember that plastic baggie of "leftover" parts?

Well here's the rub, when we as a society negate or diminish one's sense of identity, we not only set them up to fail, we set them up to die. It's like never warning people about the dangers of diabetes.

If your kid were a diabetic, you would learn every single thing you could to prevent that from happening. You would know that how you manage his/her/their diabetes at 10 years old would have a lifelong effect including their ability to complete school, get a job, have a family, food and shelter.

You would know that what you teach your child about diabetes permanently impacts their outcome in life.

You would know firsthand the pain of watching long-term dialysis and the pain of surgical procedures and rehabilitation. You would know the financial impact on your personal expenses and your insurance company (if you're lucky to have one) would know the true financial debt of that diabetes.

The harsh reality is that healthcare disparities abound for those within the LGBTQ community.

Creating health equity doesn't stop at identifying what the inequalities are, but also addressing the cause and, ultimately, the prevention.

That's the same process that created an increased awareness of diabetes. Once

Creating health equity doesn't stop at identifying what the inequalities are, but also addressing the cause and, ultimately, the prevention.

an awareness is created, society can then move toward education and prevention.

Consider that as a collective group, the LGBTQ population is at an increased risk of exposure to tobacco, alcohol, and drug use as well as high blood pressure due to increased stress and anxiety. Theresa Garnero, APRN, BC-ADM, MSN, CDE, an innovator in the field of diabetes, suggests those within the LGBTQ community have increased risks associated with diabetes. In her blog regarding Sexual Minority, *The Invisible Diabetes Disparity*, Theresa writes, "What does sexuality have to do with diabetes? A lot, according to research findings that have revealed a group of people with diabetes as large as the type 1 or gestational diabetes community. Estimates suggest that 1.3 million lesbian, gay, and bisexual (LGB) individuals have diabetes—at least 5% of the 23.6 million people with the disease in the United States."[37] This is just one of a myriad of examples the increased risk factors and complications associated with the LGBTQ identity.

For example, according to WomensHealth.gov and Healthy People 2020, lesbians, in particular, experience increased rates of obesity. Obesity is a known risk that can lead to coronary artery disease. Studies by the National Center for Biotechnology Information (NCBI) also indicate that lesbians have increased rates of high blood pressure, which can ultimately result in increased risk of stroke. In addition, according to the National LGBT Cancer Network and Healthy People 2020, lesbians have an increased rates of certain types cancers including lung, colon, and breast cancer.

The same can be said in regard to gay men for increased risks of high blood pressure and heart disease, which include

---

[37]G, T. (n.d.). The Invisible Diabetes Disparity. Retrieved February 02, 2017, from https://www.sciencedaily.com/releases/2011/05/110519090354.htm

cardiovascular and coronary artery disease, myocardial infarction (heart attacks), peripheral artery disease, and congestive heart failure according to the NCBI.

Healthy People 2020 also indicates increased rates of hepatitis B, hepatitis C, and STDs, such as HIV and HPV for gay men. The National LGBT Cancer Network reports increased rates of prostate, testicular, and colon cancer. There is also a disproportionate rate of hate crimes, victimization, depression, anxiety, bulimia, and anorexia for gay men according to Healthy People 2020.

Bisexual people tend to have higher rates of suicide attempts, intimate partner violence, obesity, eating disorders, and increased life dissatisfaction according to Healthy People 2020. Bisexual women experience higher rates of breast and ovarian cancer according to the National LGBT Cancer Network. Bisexual men also experience increased rates of intimate partner violence and depression according to Health People 2020.

To further that point, transgender people experience catastrophic consequences as discrimination (whether intentional or not) on the healthcare provider's part deters many from seeking treatment for even the most basic and preventive healthcare. In fact, the National Transgender Discrimination Survey: Report on Health and Health Care released by the National Gay and Lesbian Task Force and the National Center for Transgender Equality reports, "Nineteen percent (19%) had been refused treatment by a doctor or other provider because of their transgender or gender non-conforming status" as well as 50% of respondents reporting inadequate healthcare provider knowledge.[38] Transgender patients

---

[38]G, J. M., M, L. A., T, J., H, J. L., H, J., & K, M. (2010, October). National Transgender Discrimination Survey Report on health and health care. Retrieved February 17, 2017, from http://www.thetaskforce.org/static_html/downloads/resources_and_tools/ntds_report_on_health.pdf

are also noted to have higher rates of STDs, sexual assault, physical assault, suicide ideation and attempts, and heart disease according to Healthy People 2020.

Those within the elderly or geriatric populations of the LGBTQ community have further complications of poly-pharmacy (being prescribed multiple medications), which can be the result of lack of family interaction and/or less likely to have had children to care for them in later years. In many instances, those within the LGBTQ community have had to depend on their community family for care rather than their family of origin due to isolation and lack of social services according to the CDC.

LGTBQ youth present a completely different set of circumstances, which fuels my purpose for addressing theses issues to begin with. According to the CDC, more than 40% of LGBTQ youth have contemplated suicide and a full 29% have attempted suicide. They experience depression, increased stress, and anxiety (which is when they turn to smoking, alcohol, and drug abuse to help them cope). LGTBQ youth are five times more likely to use drugs than their heterosexual counterparts. One in 10 report missing school in the previous 30 days due to safety concerns according to the CDC. The homelessness rates, according to the *Washington Post* and the Williams Institute at UCLA Law are staggering. Reports indicate 1.6 million homeless youth each year, 40% of whom identify as LGBTQ. That's 640,000 children a year! To further put that in perspective, LGBTQ youth represent about 7% of our population.

Wait a minute, did I just say that the healthcare issues facing LGBTQ youth are depression, smoking, alcohol and drug abuse, homelessness, anxiety, and obsessive compulsive disorders?

Yep!

I didn't just contradict myself. I just illustrated that these health issues are not stereotypes but signs of ineffective coping.

That ineffective coping manifests during those adolescent years, the ones when professional help is often sought. That is the debt we pay individually and collectively for not recognizing and validating the impact of ones identity. By the time it manifests, we've missed the most valuable window of opportunity for prevention and started down on the road toward a massive collision just waiting to happen—one that ends with mass casualties including both emotional and physical implications as well as a breakdown of the family we had set out to create.

That is Identity Impact. *That* drives home the illustration that rigidly adhering to societal expectations of gender roles and identity can and does indeed have an impact on one's identity. And that impact can indeed have a lasting effect on health. That impact is experienced not only by

Rigidly adhering to societal expectations of gender roles and identity can and does indeed have an impact on one's identity.

the LGBTQ individual, but by their family, friends, and society as a whole whether it's a physical, emotional, or financial impact. Or all of the above.

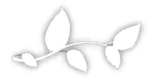

A Comparison of Life Cycles

B asic earth science 101: the life cycle of a tree begins with a seed, the formation of roots, the early growth as a seedling, a sapling, then eventually an adult, the senescent (think senior), and then decay.

Now imagine you've just been given a seed to nurture in the palm of your hand.

In order for our "seeds" to achieve self-actualization or full potential in life, we must first nurture them with physiological needs. Once those needs are met, they will feel safe and secure. That safety and security will enable them to fulfill their social needs of friendship and family which, in turn, create self-esteem, confidence, and achievement. Then they can realize self-actualization and authenticity of self—the very thing we all hope our children and loved ones will all achieve.

That safety and security will enable them to fulfill their social needs of friendship and family which, in turn, create self-esteem, confidence, and achievement.

In fact, we want this so much that we begin to plan for that from their very beginning.

Think about it, those of us who are parents began to plan for our children from the moment we knew they would arrive, maybe even before that. Through societal norms, we are ingrained to prepare for our children's arrival—prenatal visits, showers, nursery preparations (pink or blue), religious rites, etc. We've already begun to create the life we anticipate them to live.

Many of us have become so worried about meeting society's norms that we lose our own authenticity and begin to live what is expected us of versus who we are.

Never do we contemplate that as they grow and develop their own journey will be revealed to them, or how their journey will impact our own visions.

Once we complete the nursery preparations (pink or blue) and our child arrives, we move on to deciding where best to live to keep our children safe. Followed by the school years: Which school? Which district? Public? Private? We create traditions in our nuclear family and in our extended family. At the same time, we continue to meet our own social and familial pressure. All of this is then followed by academic achievement and self esteem (theirs and ours) and ultimately followed (we hope) by self-actualization—as we envision it for them (and ourselves).

Don't get me wrong, we all do it and have experienced it ourselves. The challenge is that at the top of that pyramid, that self-actualization, is *authenticity*. Many of us have become so worried about meeting society's norms that we lose our own authenticity and begin to live what is expected us of versus who we are. And we perpetuate that unknowingly in our own children and the children of others. Please don't mistake what I'm saying—expectations, norms, and mores are not bad. What I *am* saying is that we ought to be mindfully aware of the potential impact and the negation of our children's personal identity as *they* define it, and careful not to project our need to be accepted in society on our children and loved ones. Because ultimately, *they* are the ones who pay that price. And a very high price it is.

We ought to be mindfully aware of the potential impact and the negation of our children's personal identity as they define it, and careful not to project our need to be accepted in society on our children and loved ones.

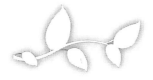

Hanging in the Balance

There is a balance between nature and nurture.

Nature, you see, is the basic or inherent feature of something, especially when seen as a characteristic of it; the living form (short, long, fat, skinny, boy, girl, etc.). Nurture is all about what we do with that gift; the process of caring for and encouraging the growth or development of someone or something.

If we are successful from the beginning, from the seed, those roots begin to form.

And, much like a tree's roots providing sustenance for growth to achieve full potential, so too, does one's identity provide sustenance and greatest growth potential.

Regardless of what society tells us our identity is—or should be—the inner core of our being knows who we are. Some of us are early bloomers and some of us are

> Much like a tree's roots providing sustenance for growth to achieve full potential, so too, does one's identity provide sustenance and greatest growth potential.

late bloomers, like myself. But all in our own time we embrace our true identities.

Ever heard the phrase "once a parent, always a parent"?

After 30 years of parenting I can honestly say that it doesn't matter how old they are, how educated they are, how financially secure they are, who they love or how many children they have, they are still my children and I still worry each and every day.

That never goes away.

Oh sure … you become more confident in their adulting skills, but when that phone rings in the middle of the night, you're immediately taken back to their high school years of worry.

Children *are* the crown on our own trees.

So where is it that we have the greatest opportunity to impact identity?

Remember that quote about expectations? "People live up to the expectations that we set." Here's a novel idea, let's change the expectation. Let's go back to the beginning with a revised instruction manual. Not just the one that tells us "What to Expect When …." but rather one that takes into account all of the parts of each of us. Not based on what society says is acceptable but rather accepting of the sum of all the parts, because that *is* the whole.

My oldest daughter (now 30) exemplifies that. Remember the show *Punky Brewster*? I used to tell her that I thought the main character was modeled after her. Punky was a saucy little thing, quick witted, somewhat snarky with her own eclectic style of clothing and hair. She had an even more individual way of looking at life. My daughter indeed lived up to that expectation then and now. And, along the way, she taught me more about what parenting meant than my own parents had. She stretched and molded my perception of myself, my role in her life, and about life in general. There's that hindsight being 20/20 again.

I wonder what knowledge I would have been able to share with her and how I could have stretched and molded her life in a more positive way had I known then what I know now about how one's identity is formed, the impact that personal identity can have on one's life, and, quite honestly, about my own identity.

How could I have more positively impacted her identity?

What I do know for sure is that nothing is worth *not* having a relationship with my children and nothing is worth risking their health and safety. I do know that I knew that to be true long before I had even an inkling that I was a lesbian myself. So much so that the thought that parents and families willingly push away those that have a differently perceived identity of themselves is foreign to me.

Before we can go back to the beginning, back to the "seed," we need to first say goodbye to the roles we hold on so tightly to. The ones based on male roles for those with male parts and female roles for those with female parts at birth.

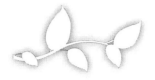

Saying Goodbye, Communicating During Grief

For those of you who have experienced loss and grief, I am truly sorry and I have great empathy for your experience. You see, as a hospice nurse and community educator, I have come to realize that both life and death are more similar in process than one would ever contemplate. In my effort to help families prepare for the final stages of life (for their loved one's final chapter), I learned to compare the giving of life to death and dying.

Many years ago, I created an in-service, an educational tool if you will, to help nursing staff and physicians feel more comfortable discussing end of life care, the ultimate goal was to help people start the conversation about the elephant in the room, to assist in opening a dialogue regarding an uncomfortable and unfamiliar yet much-needed discussion.

Not unlike the topic of communication for and with those in the LGBTQ community today.

It was in that in-service that I compared birth and living to death and dying.

Imagine the song: *I Hope You Dance* by Lee Ann Womack from 2000.

The objectives of the in-service were to:

1. Identify patient and family need for hospice intervention sooner rather than later
2. Prepare families for the inevitable changes they would face and,
3. Help them dance through their final journey

The first stage was a comparison between the confirmation of conception and the confirmation of a terminal diagnosis.

The next stage was to compare a pregnancy term of nine months and a limited life expectancy of six months or less.

The third stage was to compare symptom management to comfort. It was here that I would remind them, *"May you never take one single breath for granted."*

I would go on to discuss the commonality of spiritual changes, *"Promise me you'll give faith a fighting chance."*

Then we'd discuss anticipatory coping and planning for the changes that lie ahead, *"I hope you never fear those mountains in the distance"* as well as the emotional changes we all feel, *"Don't let some hell-bent heart leave you bitter."*

At this point, the in-service would culminate in a graphic chart comparing the stages of birth and the stages of dying, much like the one below:

Stages of Birth	Stages of Dying
Withdrawal	Withdrawal
Decreased food intake	Decreased food intake
Increased sleep	Increased sleep
Anxiety, fear	Anxiety, fear
Anticipation, uncertainty	Anticipation, uncertainty
Pain	Pain
Nausea & vomiting	Nausea & vomiting
Restlessness	Restlessness
Changes in concentration	Changes in concentration
Changes in breathing	Changes in breathing
Grunting, surge of energy	Grunting, surge of energy
Sweats & chills	Sweats & chills
Discouraged & overwhelmed	Discouraged & overwhelmed
Renewed energy	Renewed energy
Sense of elation & relief	Sense of elation & relief
Sense of closeness	Sense of closeness
Sense of detachment	Sense of detachment

I would conclude by reminding my colleagues that the main difference between giving birth and dying is the stories we share. While we share the joyful stories of being pregnant and of labor and delivery, we never talk about the other end of life. We never share that last chapter; therefore, we perceive that no one else understands what we're experiencing. We're in grief and no one else knows how we feel—or so we think.

It's at this point I would cue the end of the song, "*And when you get the choice to sit it out or dance, I hope you dance.*"

The same is true when our loved one reveals their identity. We may indeed experience grief. And it makes perfect sense, as what we perceived is no more and has never been.

How could there *not* be loss and grief? It's *how* we communicate that feeling of loss and cope with the season of change that leaves the lasting impact on both us and our loved one, whether that is our intention or not.

> It's *how* we communicate that feeling of loss and cope with the season of change that leaves the lasting impact on both us and our loved one, whether that is our intention or not.

I first learned about Elisabeth Kubler-Ross when I was in nursing school. Kubler-Ross was a Swiss-born psychiatrist and author of the 1969 ground-breaking book *On Death and Dying*. It was in this book that she first discussed the Five Stages of Grief (denial, anger, bargaining, depression, and acceptance).

In her stages of grief, Kubler-Ross initially believed that terminally ill individuals experience most of these five stages, though in no defined sequence, after being faced with the reality of their impending death. The five stages have since been adopted by many as applying to the survivors left behind and can readily be applied to loss whether in regard to physical death, loss of a pet, loss of a job, and loss of what we perceived once was.

Those emotional responses to grief can wax and wane over time.

Parents of an LGBTQ person may indeed experience Kubler-Ross's grieving process, including denial, anger, bargaining, depression, and (hopefully) acceptance. In fact, even the person themselves may experience various stages of grieving. Other family members may also grieve what they perceive they've lost.

I use the word "perceive" here but I think it's extremely important to understand, the "heartwood" or person is no different on the inside than before you (or they) came to understand their LGBTQ identity.

> It's extremely important to understand, the "heartwood" or person is no different on the inside than before you (or they) came to understand their LGBTQ identity.

Our core values as people don't change.

My personal values and beliefs, my desire to be loving, kind, and nurturing, were no different as a "heterosexual" then they are as a "lesbian."

I loved my family the same. I just came to love a part of me that had been lost in that river of denial.

I was no longer hollow on the inside. Instead, I was filled with hope.

Although my dad's journey was abbreviated and less arduous, my mother-in-law's was quite the opposite. I often find that quite poignant; you see, my wife and I had taken bets early on about who on each side of our family would be most, and least, supportive.

I envisioned my dad to respond with an eerie quiet tone, that one that makes you wait with anticipation of a loud explosion that never quite comes. Instead, what I received was a soft accepting conversation, his arms around me standing poolside. I remember his words still, "This isn't the path I would have chosen for you, from the time you were born, I envisioned your life's journey being simple and straightforward. Wishful thinking, I know, but I love you and can only imagine how challenging this is. Remember that you're not alone, I'm right beside you every step of the of way." And he has been, even when he didn't understand. Even when he feared for my safety, my health, and my decision to be a leader in my community in an effort to increase awareness and advocacy, he has loved and supported me unconditionally.

My wife, Dom, on the other hand, had envisioned her mom to be completely understanding and accepting. After all, she came out to her Mom when she was 15 years old. But her mom didn't hear her—at least it hadn't sunk in—so instead, my wife lived the life her mom had hoped for—complete with a husband, a fancy wedding, and financial security—all that was missing were the grandchildren. After a short (six-month) heterosexual marriage, Dom decided to pursue our relationship. She changed the rules of engagement. Mom wasn't happy. And she needed someone to blame—me.

It would be five years before Mom would come to accept Dom's identity.

As Dom and I learned early on in couples therapy, it takes an average of five years for a family to accept (if they ever will) their loved one's LGBTQ identity. For the most part, Dom and Mom stopped communicating. And when they did, it wasn't pretty. Little did we know Mom was keeping a journal of her thoughts and feelings (all I can say is thank goodness for Mom's therapist!)

Here's where those stages of development come back in to play.

By the time we *do* "come out" we're finally ready to live authentically. The challenge is that, just when we decide we're ready, the reality of our identity sets the grieving process for our family (that can take them *another* 5 years to come to a place of acceptance, if they ever do). Remedial math here: 5 years + 5 years = 10 years.

That's a lot of years of miscommunication or no communication at all.

Now apply that to the struggle of today's youth—by the time they "come out" they're on average 15 years old. That means 15 years minus 5 years to identify = 10 years old when they begin to question their identity.

See where I'm going with this?

Self-identification at 10 years, plus 10 years of ineffective coping for self and family, puts a child at 20 years of age. This is where those stereotypes (ineffective coping) come into play.

Here's where I share with you just how very important communication is. And the unfortunate reality that we often don't have the words to communicate our thoughts and feelings. As a result, relationships become strained, broken, and severed—not because we want them to, but because we don't have an effective means to communicate how we're feeling, what we're afraid

We often don't have the words to communicate our thoughts and feelings. As a result, relationships become strained, broken, and severed—not because we want them to, but because we don't have an effective means to communicate.

of, that we still care, and that we have no clue how to move forward with this change in the rules of engagement.

Consider Dawn:

I am 47.

I am a female heterosexual, wife, mother, teacher, Caucasian, raised Roman Catholic, but I have no belief in God. My parents have a strong faith in God and are upset that I do not attend church anymore, "after putting me through 12 years of Catholic school."

I grew up in a white, middle-class suburban neighborhood where the parental (primarily mother) expectation was to not do anything that the neighbors would question and every argument or fight could be resolved with just a "kiss and make up." My mother and father were 18 and 21, respectively, when they were married. My mother graduated from a high school where she was voted "most popular girl," class president and was head majorette of the marching band. She came from a very close-knit middle-class family, where relatives frequently visited each other. My father was the place kicker on his high school's football team. He entered the service a couple years after high school, sometime after he and my mom met. His family was on the side of lower, middle-class where no one had higher than a high school education or worked in a "career" type job (other than my father and his father). He worked very hard to provide us with a good life. He is intelligent and has a very high moral compass. My mother's family is still very close and we visit and stay in touch as much as possible.

My sister first came out to me when she was in her early 30s and I was in my mid to late 20s. I remember when she told me she was gay, she told me not to tell our parents or anyone else. She needed to tell my parents in her own way and time.

I knew she was gay, or figured as much, even before she told me. I was not shocked at all. She never had a real interest in boys or dating. Although she did have a boyfriend from time to time but was never "ga-ga" over them.

Her biggest fear was telling our parents because she knew they wouldn't take it well. They didn't at first. My mom thought it was just a stage she was going through. She was embarrassed by it and wouldn't let any of the family tell anyone else because "what would they think?"

My sister was in the convent at the time. My mother was more upset that she was leaving the convent than that she was gay. My mom had bragged for years about her daughter being a nun. In the same night my parents found out my sister was gay and leaving the convent, they also found out she was moving out of state to live with a woman she had fallen in love with. It was a lot for parents who grew up in the 40s and 50s to take in at once.

I can't speak for my sister, but I do believe she became very close friends with a couple of women she met in the convent. She was also seeing a counselor for many years to figure out "who she was." They understood her and inspired her enough to become true to herself. For my sister, our older brother probably had the most negative impact on her. He is an alcoholic and has his own self-esteem issues, which he tries to correct by talking himself up while putting others down. He said that her coming out made him drink again and leave the church. It is typical for him to blame his drinking on everyone else except himself.

For me, the person who has had the biggest impact is my sister. She is true to herself and doesn't care what others think. She made a *huge* life decision by coming out, leaving the convent, and moving across the country. She has always remained true to herself and her beliefs. Even though she left the convent, she still kept her faith in God and it even became stronger. She was the liturgist in her church and loved by the congregation. She eventually left the Catholic church because she didn't feel respected as a woman in the church as a whole. She is now a pastor of her church and a hospice chaplain. She dedicates every day of her life to helping others in need. She was the one holding my husband's hand when he died. She is married to a wonderful woman.

My mom and my sister always talked on the phone but my mom would never ask about her personal life. My sister said it was always topics about church or what my mom was doing. It wasn't until years of having to hide "the family secret" that I couldn't take it any longer and "outed" her on Facebook by posting a picture of her kissing her girlfriend. I know outing someone isn't up to anyone but the person themself. I remember feeling that my parents needed to realize that they are the minority in feeling this is wrong and it's not just a stage she was going through. My hope was to get them to understand what they were doing. She has had nothing but support from family and friends, even my mom's friends. I think most people had an inkling already anyway.

My mom has come such a *long* way with this since then. She enjoys the company of my sister's wife, talks with her on Facebook, and will ask my sister how she's doing. I think my mom realized that my sister has always been the same person with all of the wonderful qualities and morals she was raised to have. My dad still struggles with it and doesn't feel that it's right. He didn't go to my sister's wedding. But he does talk to my sister weekly and is pleasant around her wife.

My sister has seen a counselor since she was in college. I think her reason for joining the convent had a little to do with hiding her homosexuality although I'm not sure. I do believe she wanted to serve God in some way, but in the convent it didn't matter whether she was gay or straight. She could hide who she was because she had to be celibate anyway.

My sister is a strong proponent for women's rights and the rights of others, not just the LGBTQ community but anyone who is treated unjustly. Her faith is stronger because of the way her religious community embraces her as a human being.

Now, I'm not suggesting you say goodbye to anyone.

Instead, I am suggesting that, at the same time a child is progressing through those stages of development and trying to figure out their identity and role in life; parents, family and friends are progressing through their own stages of development and grieving.

I am suggesting that you take a very different look at that chart that Erik Erikson created for the stages of development.

This time, with a different set of lenses that take into account your own roots and identity, your own role in life, and how your own branches and leaves impact the roots, trunk, union graft, branches, and leaves of others. Really ponder those stages of development, not just the age-related stages, but the stages at which many

At the same time a child is progressing through those stages of development and trying to figure out their identity and role in life; parents, family and friends are progressing through their own stages of development and grieving.

Think about how the rigid sense of gender role and identity can impact the emotional, physical, educational, financial, and health outcome of each of us as individuals and as a society.

LGBQ people journey through. Think about how the rigid sense of gender role and identity can impact the emotional, physical, educational, financial, and health outcome of each of us as individuals and as a society.

I am absolutely suggesting that if you are someone providing climate and elements to others, that you do so mindfully aware of the impact that you have on the identity of others.

If you are someone providing climate and elements to others, that you do so mindfully aware of the impact that you have on the identity of others.

Is your goal to create a landscape full of indistinguishable and hollow bodies or is your goal to create a landscape of exquisite individuals full of hope?

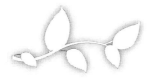

Conclusion

"Unless someone like you cares a whole awful lot,
Nothing is going to get better. It's not."

—Dr. Seuss, The Lorax

How do you and your roots, trunk, branches, and leaves impact identity?

Are you the hollow tree that breaks and causes a collision?

Or are you the tree that is full of hope, providing for other seeds and saplings the climate and culture needed to create a scenic journey we can all enjoy?

But the *biggest* question of all is:

How many of you have unwittingly driven others to that intersection?

When we project inferiority onto others, it becomes

> When we project inferiority onto others, it becomes firmly rooted in one's identity.

firmly rooted in one's identity. That sets the wheel in motion. We try to be something or someone we're not. We "fail" in our own minds, feeling that we haven't succeeded to that level that will make others love us unconditionally. We eventually resort to coping mechanisms. We feel inadequate, unworthy, unvalued, unloved, and invalid.

This is your opportunity to effect positive change and leave a lasting impact on the identity of the children of yesterday, today, and tomorrow.

This is your opportunity to effect positive change and leave a lasting impact on the identity of the children of yesterday, today, and tomorrow.

If you're a parent, I recommend considering your personal roots and biases and how they impact your child. Take some time to check out the resources at the back of this book or on my website. Talk to a trusted professional and ask how you can be a resource and support for your child as they explore their own identity, regardless of how they define it.

If you're a healthcare professional, I remind you of your commitment. Please consider taking time for self reflection of your personal roots and biases and how they may impact those you care for. How prepared are you to care for someone who identifies as LGBTQ? Take advantage of more clinical information, resources and studies provided in this book and on my website.

If you're a teacher, a counselor, or work in any profession that serves children and families, how are you bringing your roots to the landscape and what positive impact can you have?

If you are interested in more formal education for yourself or a group about the impact of identity please reach out for consulting and speaking requests.

If you are with a hospital or healthcare company with a low Human Rights Campaign (HEI) score and are interested in learning how I can help your company get to a 100, please contact me.

Additionally, if you are with a business or organization looking to hire a speaker you can visit my website for more information, DinaProto.com.

The best way to stay informed is to bookmark my website, DinaProto.com. Having been in healthcare for more than 20 years, I've accumulated a considerable amount of knowledge and insight and I look forward to cultivating conversations and growth for our present landscape.

Finally, you can connect with me online. I am on a number of social media platforms and invite you to be a part of my online network.

Connect on Facebook at: https://www.facebook.com/IdentityImpact/

Connect on LinkedIn at: https://www.linkedin.com/in/dina-proto-6b222b50/

Sign up for the monthly newsletter at: https://www.dinaproto.com/newsletter

If you have a story to share, a question to ask, or any comments, please email me at dina@dinaproto.com

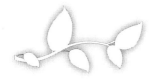

References

A Theory of Human Motivation—Abraham H Maslow—Psychological Review Vol 50 No 4 July 1943.pdf.(n.d.). Retrieved February 15, 2017, from https://docs.google.com/file/d/0B-5-JeCa2Z7hNjZlNDNh OTEtMWNkYi00YmFhLWI3YjUtMDEyMDJkZDExNWRm/edit

B, B. L., & R, K. A. (n.d.). Analysis of LGBT Identity Development Models and Implications for Practice. Retrieved February 02, 2017, from https://msu.edu/~renn./BilodeauRennNDSS.pdf

Complication. (n.d.). Retrieved March 15, 2017, from https://www.merriam-webster.com/dictionary/complication#medicalDictionary

Dan Gill, The Times-Picayune garden columnist. (2015, March 05). How, when and why plants are grafted. Retrieved April 18, 2017, from http://www.nola.com/homegarden/index.ssf/2015/03/how_when_and_why_plants_are_gr.html

Disparities. (n.d.). Retrieved March 15, 2017, from https://www.healthypeople.gov/2020/about/foundation-health-measures/Disparities

Forcing Kids To Stick To Gender Roles Can Actually Be Harmful To Their Health. (n.d.). Retrieved April 20, 2017, from https://thinkprogress.org/forcing-kids-to-stick-to-gender-roles-can-actually-be-harmful-to-their-health-34aef42199f2

G, J. M., M, L. A., T, J., H, J. L., H, J., & K, M. (2010, October). National Transgender Discrimination Survey Report on health and health care. Retrieved February 17, 2017, from http://www.thetaskforce.

org/static_html/downloads/resources_and_tools/ntds_report_on_health.pdf

G, T. (n.d.). The Invisible Diabetes Disparity. Retrieved February 02, 2017, from https://www.sciencedaily.com/releases/2011/05/11051 9090354.htm

Gallup, I. (2017, January 11). In US, More Adults Identifying as LGBT. Retrieved April 18, 2017, from http://www.gallup.com/poll/201731/lgbt-identification-rises.aspx?g_source=Social Issues& g_medium=newsfeed&g_campaign=tiles

Gates, G. J. (2011, April). How many people are lesbian, gay, bisexual and transgender? . Retrieved April, 2017, from https://williamsinstitute.law.ucla.edu/wp-content/uploads/Gates-How-Many-People-LGBT-Apr-2011.pdf

Gender Identity Development in Children. (n.d.). Retrieved April 17, 2017, from https://www.healthychildren.org/English/ages-stages/gradeschool/Pages/Gender-Identity-and-Gender-Confusion-In-Children.aspx

Growth ring. (2017, August 11). Retrieved September 03, 2017, from https://simple.wikipedia.org/wiki/Growth_ring

H, K. (2007, March). Models that Change: The Study of Gay Identity Development. Retrieved February 02, 2017, from https://dspace.ucalgary.ca/bitstream/1880/47539/1/Heng_2007.pdf

Hunt, J. (n.d.). Why the Gay and Transgender Population Experiences Higher Rates of Substance Use. Retrieved March 25, 2017, from https://www.americanprogress.org/issues/lgbt/reports/2012/03/09/11228/why-the-gay-and-transgender-population-experiences-higher-rates-of-substance-use/

Identity Status Theory (Marcia). (2016, September 03). Retrieved March 15, 2017, from https://www.learning-theories.com/identity-status-theory-marcia.html

Identity. (n.d.). Retrieved March 16, 2017, from https://www.merriam-webster.com/dictionary/identity

Identity. (n.d.). Retrieved March 16, 2017, from https://www.merriam-webster.com/dictionary/identity#medicalDictionary

Institute of Medicine (US) Committee on Lesbian, Gay, Bisexual, and Transgender Health Issues and Research Gaps and Opportunities. The Health of Lesbian, Gay, Bisexual, and Transgender People: Building a Foundation for Better Understanding. Washington (DC): National Academies Press (US); 2011. 4, Childhood/Adolescence. Available from: https://www.ncbi.nlm.nih.gov/books/NBK64808/ Lesbian, Gay, Bisexual, and Transgender Health. (n.d.). Retrieved April 18, 2017, from https://www.healthypeople.gov/2020/topics-objectives/ topic/lesbian-gay-bisexual-and-transgender-health

Lytle, M. C., Vaughan, M. D., Rodriguez, E. M., & Shmerler, D. L. (2014, October 01). Working with LGBT Individuals: Incorporating Positive Psychology into Training and Practice. Retrieved February 15, 2017, from https://www.ncbi.nlm.nih.gov/pmc/articles/PMC4276565/

MA, J. W. (2016, April 01). News and Internet Searches About HIV After Celebrity Disclosure. Retrieved February 28, 2017, from http://jamanetwork.com/journals/jamainternalmedicine/fullarticle/2495274

McLeod, S. (1970, January 01). Erikson's Psychosocial Stages of Development. Retrieved April 20, 2017, from https://www.simplypsychology.org/Erik-Erikson.html

Mitchell, T. (2016, September 28). 5. Vast majority of Americans know someone who is gay, fewer know someone who is transgender. Retrieved April 18, 2017, from http://www.pewforum.org/2016/09/28/5-vast-majority-of-americans-know-someone-who-is-gay-fewer-know-someone-who-is-transgender/

Sentinel event. (2017, August 20). Retrieved September 15, 2017, from https://en.wikipedia.org/wiki/Sentinel_event

Serving Our Youth 2015: The Needs and Experiences of Lesbian, Gay, Bisexual, Transgender, and Questioning Youth Experiencing Homelessness. (2015, June 05). Retrieved February 15, 2017, from https://williamsinstitute.law.ucla.edu/research/safe-schools-and-youth/serving-our-youth-2015-the-needs-and-experiences-of-lesbian-gay-bisexual-transgender-and-questioning-youth-experiencing-homelessness/

Sign. (n.d.). Retrieved March 15, 2017, from https://www.merriam-webster.com/dictionary/sign#medicalDictionary

Symptom. (n.d.). Retrieved March 15, 2017, from https://www.merriam-webster.com/dictionary/symptom#medicalDictionary

The Anatomy of a Tree. (2002, February 27). Retrieved March 15, 2017, from http://www.sactree.com/assets/files/greenprint/toolkit/c/huntsvilleTreeGuide.pdf

"What's in Store: Moving Away from Gender-Based Signs." Target Corporate, corporate.target.com/article/2015/08/gender-based-signs-corporate. Accessed 18 Apr. 2017.

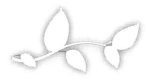

Resources

American Academy of Pediatrics
https://www.aap.org/en-us/about-the-aap/Committees-Councils-Sections/solgbt/Pages/informationforfamilies.aspx

American Cancer Society
https://www.cancer.org/healthy/find-cancer-early/womens-health/cancer-facts-for-lesbians-and-bisexual-women.html

Campus Pride
https://www.campuspride.org

Centers for Disease Control
https://www.cdc.gov/lgbthealth/

Community Marketing Inc.
https://communitymarketinginc.com

Dina Proto, RN
http://www.dinaproto.com

Diversity Best Practices
https://diversitybestpractices.com

Family Equality Council
http://www.familyequality.org

Fenway
http://fenwayhealth.org/the-fenway-institute/

Gay and Lesbian Medical Association
http://www.glma.org

GLAAD
https://www.glaad.org

GLSEN
https://www.glsen.org

GSA Network
https://gsanetwork.org/sexualhealth

Healthy Children in Association with the American Academy of
Pediatrics
https://www.healthychildren.org/English/ages-stages/Pages/
default.aspx

Healthy Children in Association with the American Academy of
Pediatrics
https://www.HealthyChildren.org

Healthy People Initiatives
https://www.cdc.gov/nchs/healthy_people/index.htm

InterAct Advocates
https://interactadvocates.org

Lambda Legal
https://www.lambdalegal.org

LGBTQ Population Siza Data (Gallup poll)
https://gallup.com/poll/201731/lgbt-identification-rises.aspx

Matthew Shepard Foundation
https://www.matthewshepard.org/about-us/

National Association of LGBTQ Journalists
https://www.nlgja.org

National Association of Addiction Professionals
https://www.nalgap.org

National Center for Transgender Equality
https://www.transequality.org

National Coalition for LGBT Health
https://healthlgbt.org/about-us/

National Gay and Lesbian Chamber of Commerce
https://www.nglcc.org

National LGBT Cancer Network
https://cancer-network.org

National LGBT Health Education Centerhttps://www.lgbthealth
education.org/lgbt-education/lgbt-health-resources/

National LGBT Tobacco Control Network
https://www.lgbttobacco.org

Out & Equal Workplace Advocates
https://outandequal.org

Parents, Families, Friends and Loved Ones of Lesbians and Gays
https://www.pflag.org

Substance Abuse and Mental Health Services Association
https://store.samhsa.gov/shin/content/SMA12-4684/
SMA12-4684.pdf

Teazled Greeting Cards & Gifts
https://www.teazled.com

The Trevor Project
https://www.thetrevorproject.org

The Williams Institute UCLA Law
https://williamsinstitute.law.ucla.edu

Transgender Law Center
https://transgenderlawcenter.org

True Colors
https://truecolorsfund.org/our-issue/

Tyler Clementi Foundation
https://tylerclementi.org

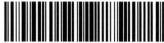

Made in the USA
Columbia, SC
06 December 2017